Neurotology

What Do I Do Now?

SERIES CO-EDITORS-IN-CHIEF

Lawrence C. Newman, MD
Director of the Headache Institute
Department of Neurology
St. Luke's Hospital Center
New York, NY

Morris Levin, MD
Co-director of the Dartmouth Headache Center
Director of the Dartmouth Neurology Residency Training Program
Section of Neurology
Dartmouth Hitchcock Medical Center
Lebanon, NH

PREVIOUS VOLUMES IN THE SERIES

Headache and Facial Pain
Peripheral Nerve and Muscle Disease
Pediatric Neurology
Stroke
Epilepsy
Neurocritical Care
Neuro-Ophthalmology
Neuroimmunology
Pain
Neuroinfections
Emergency Neurology
Cerebrovascular Disease
Movement Disorders
Neurogenetics

Neurotology

Darius Kohan, MD
Director of Otology/Neurotology
Lenox Hill Hospital and Manhattan Eye Ear Nose and Throat Hospital, NJ/LIJ
Associate Professor of Otolaryngology
New York University Medical School
President of the New York Otologic Society
Board of Governors, New York Otologic Society
New York, NY

Selena E. Heman-Ackah, MD, MBA
Director of Otology, Neurotology and Audiology
Division of Otolaryngology, Head and Neck Surgery
Beth Israel Deaconess Medical Center
Harvard Medical School
Boston, MA

Sujana S. Chandrasekhar, MD, FACS
Director, New York Otology
Director of the Comprehensive Balance Center of the New York Head and Neck Institute
Clinical Associate Professor of Otolaryngology
Mount Sinai School of Medicine
New York, NY

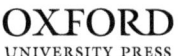

OXFORD
UNIVERSITY PRESS

Oxford University Press is a department of the University of Oxford.
It furthers the University's objective of excellence in research,
scholarship, and education by publishing worldwide.

Oxford New York
Auckland Cape Town Dar es Salaam Hong Kong Karachi
Kuala Lumpur Madrid Melbourne Mexico City Nairobi
New Delhi Shanghai Taipei Toronto

With offices in
Argentina Austria Brazil Chile Czech Republic France Greece
Guatemala Hungary Italy Japan Poland Portugal Singapore
South Korea Switzerland Thailand Turkey Ukraine Vietnam

Oxford is a registered trademark of Oxford University Press
in the UK and certain other countries.

Published in the United States of America by
Oxford University Press
198 Madison Avenue, New York, NY 10016

© Oxford University Press 2014

All rights reserved. No part of this publication may be reproduced, stored in a
retrieval system, or transmitted, in any form or by any means, without the prior
permission in writing of Oxford University Press, or as expressly permitted by law,
by license, or under terms agreed with the appropriate reproduction rights organization.
Inquiries concerning reproduction outside the scope of the above should be sent to the
Rights Department, Oxford University Press, at the address above.

You must not circulate this work in any other form
and you must impose this same condition on any acquirer.

Library of Congress Cataloging-in-Publication Data
Kohan, Darius, 1959– author.
Neurotology / Darius Kohan, Selena Heman-Ackah, Sujana Chandrasekhar.
  p. ; cm.
Includes bibliographical references.
ISBN 978-0-19-984398-5 (alk. paper)
I. Heman-Ackah, Selena, author. II. Chandrasekhar, Sujana S., author. III. Title.
[DNLM: 1. Nervous System Diseases—Case Reports. 2. Otorhinolaryngologic
Diseases—Case Reports. 3. Neurotology—methods—Case Reports. WV 140]
RC346
616.8—dc23
2014005477

The science of medicine is a rapidly changing field. As new research and clinical experience broaden our
knowledge, changes in treatment and drug therapy occur. The author and publisher of this work have
checked with sources believed to be reliable in their efforts to provide information that is accurate and
complete, and in accordance with the standards accepted at the time of publication. However, in light of
the possibility of human error or changes in the practice of medicine, neither the author, nor the publisher,
nor any other party who has been involved in the preparation or publication of this work warrants that the
information contained herein is in every respect accurate or complete. Readers are encouraged to confirm
the information contained herein with other reliable sources, and are strongly advised to check the product
information sheet provided by the pharmaceutical company for each drug they plan to administer.

Acknowledgments

To Mr. Joseph Agosta and Mr. Jonathan Komisar, whose able assistance with image procurement makes this text all the more valuable for the reader.

Preface

My father, Silviu Kohan, a wise physician to whom I dedicate this book, always emphasized to medical students and residents the importance of cooperating with their colleagues in a multidisciplinary approach in order to optimize patient care. His advice is most appropriate when managing patients with complex neurologic/neurotologic signs and symptoms with an extensive differential diagnosis and treatment options.

In this text we provide a general overview of common and important neurotologic pathology, and present real cases we all managed at our institutions. The focus is on hearing loss, tinnitus, vertigo/dysequilibrium, facial neuropathy, and neurologic complications of otitis media. In each section an attempt was made to provide a clear diagnostic protocol and appropriate therapeutic modalities for each neurotologic pathology under consideration. Current controversies involving the diagnostic evaluation and treatment options mentioned in the text are reviewed in much greater detail in the "Further Reading" component of each chapter.

The authors are very grateful to two key individuals, Mr. Joseph Michael Agosta and Mr. Jonathan Komisar, MS, who provided invaluable aid in the production of this manuscript. We also thank Lawrence Newman, MD, Mr. Craig Panner, and Ms. Marni Rolfes for promoting this project to fruition. Most of all we want to thank you, the reader, for taking care of patients with neurotologic disorders, which one day could be any one of us.

Darius Kohan, MD
Associate Professor, NYU School of Medicine
Director of Otology/Neurotology-Lenox Hill/MEETH Medical Center

Table of Contents

SECTION I HEARING LOSS

1 **Presbycusis** 3
Darius Kohan
With the population older than age 65 years being the largest growing age-group in the United States, the prevalence of presbycusis is on the rise. Presbycusis is characterized by high-frequency sensorineural hearing loss and occasionally with deficits in central auditory processing. This chapter reviews the pathogenesis of presbycusis, the diagnostic evaluation, and current available treatment modalities.

2 **Sudden Sensorineural Hearing Loss** 13
Darius Kohan
Sudden sensorineural hearing loss is a condition commonly encountered in the neurologic and neurotologic practice. The potential etiology, diagnostic evaluation, and treatment of sudden sensorineural hearing loss are discussed.

3 **Noise-Induced Hearing Loss** 21
Darius Kohan
The incidence of noise-induced hearing loss is increasing. It is characterized by high-frequency sensorineural hearing loss with associated nonpulsatile tinnitus. This chapter reviews the OSHA guidelines for noise exposure, and the phases of noise-induced hearing loss are described. Additionally, the evaluation, treatment, and prevention of noise-induced hearing loss are discussed.

4 **Ototoxins** 27
Darius Kohan
Ototoxin exposure is a common cause or contributing factor in the pathogenesis of sensorineural hearing loss. This chapter reviews commonly encountered ototoxins and potential means for reducing effects of ototoxic agents.

5 **Congenital Hearing Loss** 33
Darius Kohan
Congenital hearing loss can be characterized as sensorineural, conductive, or mixed hearing loss. Additionally, congenital hearing loss can be classified as syndromic or nonsyndromic. This chapter reviews the classification of congenital hearing loss and its associated differential. The diagnostic evaluation and management of congenital hearing loss are discussed.

6 **Neurofibromatosis** 39
Darius Kohan
The two types of neurofibromatosis are both associated with hearing loss and tinnitus and are autosomal-dominant. They have distinct presentation and different clinicopathology. The etiology, diagnostic work-up, and treatment options are reviewed.

7 **Vestibular Schwannomas and Menigiomas** 45
Darius Kohan
Vestibular schwannomas are the most common lesions of the cerebellopontine angle and represent about 6–8% of all intracranial tumors. Meningiomas are the most common intracranial neoplasms accounting for about 20% of lesions; however, they are second to acoustic neuromas at the CPA. The pathophysiology, diagnostic work up and therapeutic options are discussed in detail. Audiovestibular tests and imaging modalities are necessary. Therapy is based on patient age and medical status, tumor size, neurologic deficits and may involve observation, stereotactic surgery, or surgery either for tumor decompression of complete excision. Complications of therapy including facial nerve injury, hearing loss, and other neurologic deficits are address in the text concurrent with possible corrective modalities.

8 **Rare Tumors of the Cerebellopontine Angle** 55
Darius Kohan
The differential for tumors involving the cerebellopontine angle (CPA) can be quite extensive. Although meningiomas are the most common intracranial tumors, vestibular schwannoma (also known as acoustic neuroma), are the most common tumor of the CPA and account for 8% of all intracranial tumors. The clinical presentation of CPA tumors, including asymmetric hearing loss and dysequilibrium, is reviewed. The differential for cerebellopontine angle tumors, characteristic findings on magnetic resonance imaging and computed tomography imaging, and potential treatments are discussed.

SECTION II   VERTIGO AND DYSEQUILIBRIUM

9 **Ménière's Disease** 65
Selena E. Heman-Ackah
Ménière's disease is characterized by episodic vertigo, tinnitus, and fluctuating hearing lasting minutes to hours. Its etiology is thought to be secondary to endolymphatic hydrops. The diagnostic evaluation and graduated treatment modalities are reviewed. The natural history of Ménière's disease is also discussed.

10 Vestibular Neuropathy 75
Selena E. Heman-Ackah
Vestibular neuropathy is characterized by constant vertigo, dysequilibrium, nausea, and vomiting without associated hearing loss, which lasts for approximately days to 1 week. The clinical presentation, diagnosis, and treatment of vestibular neuropathy are discussed.

11 Labyrinthitis 83
Selena E. Heman-Ackah
Labyrinthitis is a common cause of vertigo. It is characterized by vertigo and unilateral hearing loss lasting approximately days to 1 week. The presence of associated hearing loss helps in distinguishing this diagnosis from vestibular neuropathy. The clinical presentation, diagnosis, and treatment for labyrinthitis are discussed in this chapter.

12 Benign Paroxysmal Positional Vertigo 91
Selena E. Heman-Ackah
Benign paroxysmal positional vertigo (BPPV) is caused by displacement of otolith. It is characterized by vertigo lasting seconds following head position change. The Dix-Hallpike maneuver reveals fatigable rotary nystagmus, which is pathognomonic for BPPV. The clinical presentation, diagnosis, and treatment of BPPV including otolith repositioning therapy are discussed.

13 Migrainous Vertigo 97
Selena E. Heman-Ackah
Vertigo in association with migraine is a recently identified entity. Patients with migraine-associated vertigo often report history of vertigo without associated headache making the diagnosis challenging. This chapter reviews the diagnostic criteria for migraine-associated vertigo as well as its management.

14 Perilymphatic Fistula 105
Selena E. Heman-Ackah
Perilymphatic fistula may occur at either the round or oval window. It is associated with vertigo exacerbated by the Valsalva maneuver or straining. Similarly, exposure to loud noise can precipitate vertigo. Its etiology is most often traumatic; there is controversy regarding an idiopathic, spontaneous etiology. The controversies regarding the etiology of perilymphatic fistula along with its characteristic presentation, diagnostic evaluation, and treatment are discussed.

15 Superior Semicircular Canal Dehiscence 113
Selena E. Heman-Ackah
Superior semicircular canal dehiscence (SSCD) is a recently identified entity associated with vertigo. Like perilymphatic fistula, SSCD presents with

vertigo in association with strain and the Valsalva maneuver. True, fine-cut, coronal computed tomography imaging of the temporal bone is critical to the diagnosis of SCCD. In this chapter, the presenting symptoms, clinical evaluation, diagnostic work-up, and treatment of SCCD are discussed.

16 **Labyrinthine Concussion** 123
Selena E. Heman-Ackah
Posttraumatic vertigo is commonly encountered. The differential for posttraumatic vertigo is significant including benign paroxysmal positional vertigo, perilymphatic fistula, and posttraumatic Ménière's disease (or endolymphatic hydrops), which have been addressed in previous chapters. Labyrinthine concussion is included within the differential of posttraumatic vertigo. This chapter reviews the clinical presentation, diagnostic evaluation, and treatment of labyrinthine concussion.

SECTION III TINNITUS

17 **Subjective Tinnitus** 133
Sujana S. Chandrasekhar
The differential diagnosis for subjective tinnitus is vast. This chapter describes the differential diagnosis of subjective tinnitus. The diagnostic evaluation and treatment of subjective tinnitus are also discussed.

18 **Paragangliomas** 143
Sujana S. Chandrasekhar
Paragangliomas (also known as glomus tumors) are benign neuroendocrine tumors. Glomus tympanicum and glomus jugulare are tumors that present in the temporal bone with pulsatile tinnitus, conductive hearing loss, and cranial nerve neuropathy. Further description of the origin of these tumors, their clinical presentation, diagnostic evaluation, and options for treatment are discussed.

19 **Arteriovenous Malformations, Arteriovenous Fistulas, and Aberrant Vasculature** 151
Sujana S. Chandrasekhar
Arteriovenous malformations and aberrant vasculature of the temporal bone are often associated with the presentation of pulsatile tinnitus. The embryology, etiology, diagnosis, and management of these challenging lesions of the temporal bone are discussed in detail.

20 **Benign Intracranial Hypertension** 159
Sujana S. Chandrasekhar
Benign intracranial hypertension is a relatively common etiology of tinnitus, often pulsatile, and associated with numerous other neurologic findings. The etiology, presentation, diagnosis, and management are discussed.

21 **Tegmen Dehiscence, Including Superior Semicircular Canal Dehiscence** 163
Sujana S. Chandrasekhar
Dehiscence of the tegmen tympani or mastoidium is often associated with pulsatile tinnitus. The etiology of tegmen dehiscence is discussed in this chapter. The diagnosis and management are also reviewed.

SECTION IV FACIAL NEUROPATHY

22 **Congenital Facial Palsy** 169
Selena E. Heman-Ackah
The differential diagnosis for congenital facial palsy is reviewed. The diagnostic evaluation and management options for congenital facial palsy are also discussed.

23 **Bell's Palsy** 175
Selena E. Heman-Ackah
Bell's palsy or idiopathic facial paresis is a diagnosis of exclusion. The etiology of Bell's palsy is believed to be viral. A differential for facial paralysis including Lyme disease and Ramsay Hunt syndrome are discussed. Diagnostic evaluation of facial paralysis and the management and natural history of Bell's palsy are reviewed.

24 **Traumatic Facial Palsy** 183
Selena E. Heman-Ackah
Facial palsy is commonly encountered in temporal bone (TB) trauma. In this chapter, the etiology of facial palsy in trauma is discussed. The diagnostic evaluation and classification of TB trauma, longitudinal versus transverse and otic-capsule involving versus otic-sparing TB fractures are reviewed in the context of hearing loss and facial palsy. The management of posttraumatic facial palsy is reviewed.

25 **Facial Neuroma** 193
Selena E. Heman-Ackah
Facial neuroma commonly presents with facial paresis and hearing loss. It is essential to differentiate facial neuroma from vestibular schwannoma. This chapter reviews the clinical presentation and diagnostic evaluation of facial neuroma as well as available treatment options and complications thereof.

SECTION V NEUROLOGIC COMPLICATIONS OF OTITIS MEDIA

26 **Facial Paralysis** 201
   Sujana S. Chandrasekhar
   The first complication of otitis media to be reviewed is facial paralysis. A description of the diagnostic evaluation and treatment of otitis media complicated by facial paralysis are discussed.

27 **Petrous Apicitis** 207
   Sujana S. Chandrasekhar
   Gradenigo's triad of abducens palsy, retro-orbital pain, and suppurative otitis media are characteristic findings of petrous apicitis. The clinical presentation, diagnosis, and treatment of petrous apicitis are reviewed.

28 **Meningitis and Brain Abscess** 211
   Sujana S. Chandrasekhar
   Fatigue, malaise, nuchal rigidity, and mental status changes are alarming findings in the patient with otitis media. Meningitis secondary to otitis media is relatively uncommon. Brain abscess is an even less commonly encountered complication of otitis media. However, when present the sequelae of meningitis and brain abscess can be devastating. Swift diagnosis and effective treatment are critical. The diagnosis, treatment, and associated morbidity of meningitis and brain abscess secondary to otitis media are discussed.

29 **Otitic Hydrocephalus** 217
   Sujana S. Chandrasekhar
   Otic hydrocephalus is an uncommon complication of otitis media. It is characterized by increased intracranial pressure without associated hydrocephalus. Patients present with headache, malaise, and vision changes. Papilledema and abducens palsy on ocular examination are common clinical finding. The presentation, clinical evaluation, and management of otic hydrocephalus are discussed.

30 **Lateral or Sigmoid Sinus Thrombosis** 221
   Sujana S. Chandrasekhar
   Lateral sinus and sigmoid sinus thrombosis are rare complications of otitis media that often present with picket fence fevers and signs of sepsis. The clinical presentation, diagnostic evaluation, management, and complications are reviewed.

Index 227

SECTION I

Hearing Loss

1 Presbycusis

A 68-year-old female piano teacher noticed increasing bilateral hearing loss (HL) and nonpulsatile fluctuating tinnitus. The tinnitus is most bothersome in the morning and is better during the day. The HL is worse on the left. She has no otalgia, otorrhea, vertigo, disequilibrium, or history of head trauma. She has difficulty appreciating music concerts and operas. Her father had HL with aging. Her mother was diagnosed with transient ischemic attacks and HL before a devastating cerebrovascular accident. Because she is afraid of developing a "stroke" she takes a baby aspirin daily for about 5 years. The rest of her past medical history is unremarkable. The physical examination is normal. On tuning fork tests, the Weber is midline and Rinne is normal with air better than bone conduction. The audiogram (Figure 1-1) reveals bilateral symmetrical sloping moderately severe sensorineural HL (SNHL) with normal speech discrimination scores and tympanogram.

What do you do now?

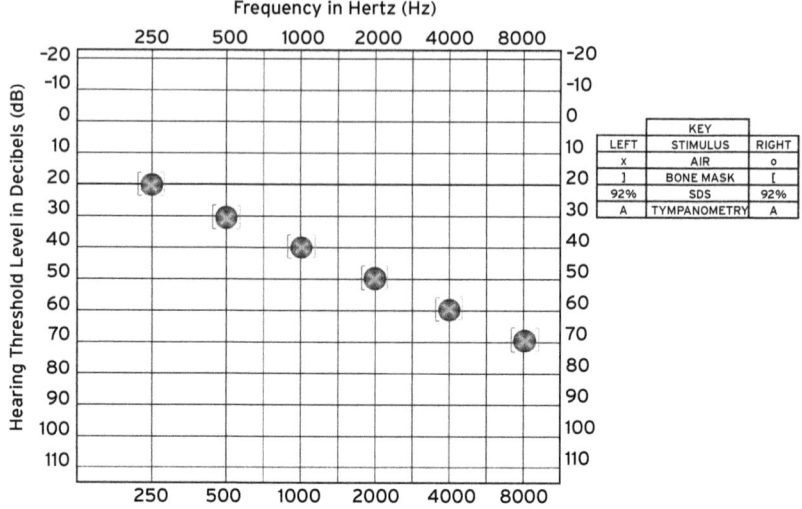

FIGURE 1-1 Audiogram reveals a bilateral symmetric sloping moderately-severe sensorineural hearing Loss (SNHL).

Presbycusis is progressive SNHL associated with aging. About 30% of people 65–70 years old and more than 50% of those 75 years and older in the United States have significant HL. Up to 3% of the U.S. population may benefit from amplification devices. Longitudinal studies on HL correlating to age, sex, and noise exposure reveal that 97% of people experience HL with aging. If younger than 55 years old the average is 3 dB HL per decade and if older than 55 years, 9 dB HL per decade. In general older patients also have worse speech discrimination relative to younger patients with the same level of hearing acuity consistent with deficits in neural processing and end-organ pathology. Decreased neural cell population and increasing synaptic time in central processing in combination with diminished ability to detect interaural time differences result in poorer hearing, worse discrimination, and worse localization of speech. The entire auditory pathway deteriorates with age, as documented by serial otoacoustic emission (OAE) and auditory brainstem response (ABR) studies with deterioration noted at the level of the superior olivary complex, lateral lemniscus, inferior colliculus, and the more proximal cochlear nucleus.[1]

Throughout life, acoustic trauma, genetic preprogrammed senescence, mitochondrial gene mutations, cardiovascular disease, metabolic disorders, nutrition, and ototoxic substance exposure all play a role in the multifactorial etiology of presbycusis. The HL is usually symmetrical, more prominent in the high frequencies, and usually more severe in males, the last probably caused by sociocultural lifestyle behavior. Peripheral pathology is documented by decreasing OAE with age.[1-3]

There are four major types of presbycusis[1,3] based on histopathology (Table 1-1):

1. Sensory: Bilateral(AU) symmetric abruptly sloping high-frequency HL. Beginning in middle age, there is loss of both hair cells (outer more than inner) and decrease in supporting sustentacular cells at the basal turn of the cochlea with lipofuscin deposition in the hair cells and loss of stereocilia. Speech discrimination is usually good.
2. Neural: Loss of spiral ganglion cells; average loss is 2100 out of total 35,000 neurons per decade. Over 50% neuronal loss is required for detectable HL. The loss in speech discrimination is relatively more severe than with sensory HL and corresponds to more neuronal loss in the apical cochlea (lower frequencies). The downward sloping audiometric pattern is more variable.
3. Strial: HL is typically flat on audiogram with relatively good discrimination. The metabolically active stria vascularis degenerates and the secretion of endolymph and homeostasis of

TABLE 1-1 **Characteristics of Hearing Loss in Presbycusis**

Type	Pure Tones	Speech Discrimination
Sensory	High tones, abrupt slope	Related to frequencies lost
Neural	All frequencies; variable pattern	Severe loss
Strial	All frequencies	Minimal loss
Cochlear conductive	High tones, gradual slope	Related to steepness of high-tone loss

Source: Lalwani AK. The aging inner ear. In: Anil K. Lalwani, editor. Current Diagnosis and Treatment in Otolaryngology-Head and Neck Surgery. Lange Medical Books/McGraw-Hill, New York, NY, 2004. pp. 735–42.

ionic potentials is reduced resulting in progressive HL. Atrophy may involve the entire cochlea.
4. Conductive/Mechanical: Increasing mechanical stiffness of basilar membrane and cochlear duct is hypothesized to produce a gradual sloping high-frequency SNHL with progressively worse discrimination. No definitive histologic correlate has been documented.

Among patients with bilateral (AU) severe-to-profound SNHL with disproportionate poor speech discrimination, 6% have normal OAE and cochlear microphonics implying normal outer hair cell function in the organ of Corti. These patients with AU pure SNHL have severely abnormal ABR starting at wave I (the acoustic nerve) and are diagnosed with auditory neuropathy.[4,5] A genetic predisposition is present in about 40% of these patients; however, in most there is no identifiable cause for the HL. Metabolic abnormalities, infection, and immunologic defects may contribute to this condition. The temporal bone computer tomography and brain magnetic resonance imaging (MRI) are normal in patients with auditory neuropathy. Functional MRI may in the future help identify a more specific pathology. The most likely pathophysiology is desynchrony of the auditory pathways, possibly caused by demyelination. About 75% of patients with auditory neuropathy are younger than age 10. The configuration of the audiogram varies frequently and changes with time in most of these patients; however, the common denominator is always disproportionately poor speech discrimination. Approximately 80% of adult patients with auditory neuropathy may also have other peripheral neuropathies, thus nerve conduction studies may help. If positive, a subsequent sural nerve biopsy is confirmatory of concurrent peripheral neuropathy. These patients do not usually have any vestibular symptoms, thus vestibular tests are not necessary. Because of poor speech discrimination, amplification often fails to rehabilitate the auditory deficit. However, cochlear implants, which restore neural synchrony, are most useful.[6]

The patient presented here has a long history of music exposure (not necessarily loud) as a music teacher. The audiogram is more consistent with sensory presbycusis. The only work-up needed after the history and physical examination was the audiogram. Often patients with presbycusis have tinnitus in a quiet environment, sometimes severe enough to cause insomnia. Tinnitus treatment is discussed in a later section in this book. The feeling that the HL is asymmetrical, even though the audiogram does not document this, is very common and no further testing is required. Fluctuations in eustachian tube function and external ear pathology are the most common etiologies for feeling of asymmetry.

The social withdrawal associated in the elderly with auditory deficits must be addressed promptly to avoid further mental status deterioration.[5] Treatment consists of appropriate aural habilitation, such as hearing aids, assistive-listening devices (television headphones, telecoils, FM systems, telephone amplifiers, TTY, and so forth), implantable bone conduction hearing processors (BAHA/Ponto/Sophono), implantable middle ear auditory processors (e.g., Vibrant Soundbridge, Envoy/Esteem system), or cochlear implants. The listening environment must be modified to optimize clarity and diminish background noise. Lip reading education occasionally helps.[5,7]

Hearing aids are now of exceptional high quality. They are cosmetic unobtrusive digital programmable microprocessors with directional microphones, telecoils, and frequency-specific capabilities to amplify desired sounds while dampening noise depending on the acoustic environment. Regardless of the severity of the HL and the speech discrimination, all patients derive some benefit (auditory or tactile) from proper amplification. There is enhanced audition and localization of sound. Hearing aid recommendations are individualized; however, in general they are indicated for patients with speech reception threshold higher than 25 dB and/or speech discrimination scores lower than 80% if word presentation is at normal conversation level of 50 dB.[7]

Implantable hearing processors and bone conduction devices are best used in patients who have outer or middle ear pathology preventing the use of standard hearing aids. The sound is transmitted by bone conduction either directly to the cochlea or via a vibrating ossicle attachment device, such as the Vibrant floating mass transducer (Figure 1-2), a bone-anchored hearing aid processor (Figure 1-3), the SoundBite device (Figure 1-4), or the Sophono system (Figure 1-5).[8,9]

Cochlear implants, until recently, were only indicated in patients with bilateral severe to profound HL and poor discrimination where standard amplification is inadequate. In February, 2014 the FDA approved these

1. Sounds are picked up by the microphone of the audio processor. The audio processor is held over the implant by magnetic attraction to a magnet in the implanted part.

2. The audio processor converts sounds into electrical signals.

3. These signals are transmitted across the skin to the implant.

4. The implant relays the signal further to the FMT (Floating Mass Transducer). The FMT is the core component of the system and is smaller than a grain of rice.

5. The FMT converts the signal into machanical vibrations that directly drive a middle ear structure (e.g. the ossicular chain) and cause it to vibrate.

6. These vibrations then conduct sound to the inner ear and on to the brain where they are perceived as sound.

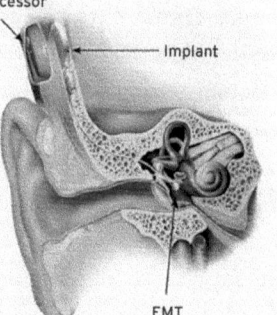

FIGURE 1-2 The Vibrant Soundbridge Middke Ear Implant. Image courtesy of VIBRANT MED-EL Hearing Technology GmbH.

(a)

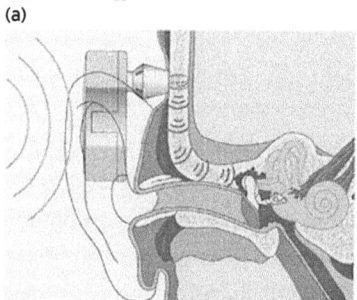

Sound waves travelling in the inner ear

(b)

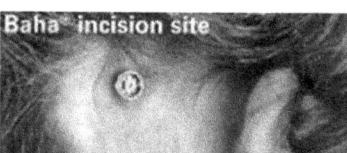

FIGURE 1-3 (a) BAHA System: Clip-on auditory processor sends sound vibrations to the surgically implanted abutment-screw-fixture complex which transmits sound waves to the cochlea. (b) BAHA Abutment Site- skin site where auditory processor is attached. Images courtesy of Cochlear Americas.

(a)

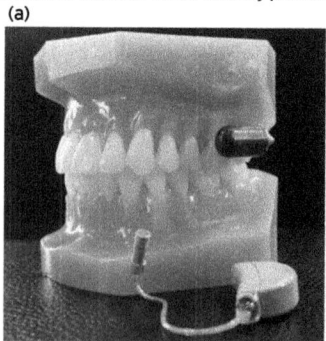

(b)

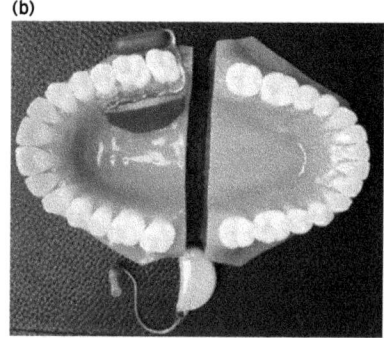

FIGURE 1-4 SoundBite Hearing System. (a) closed bite view and (b) open bite view- demonstrate In-the Mouth (ITM) hearing device and the Behind-the-Ear (BTE) microphone unit. The ITM processor transmits the sound waves picked up by the ear level microphone to the teeth which vibrate and conduct the sound via skull bones to the cochlea. Models courtesy of Sonitus Medical, INC.

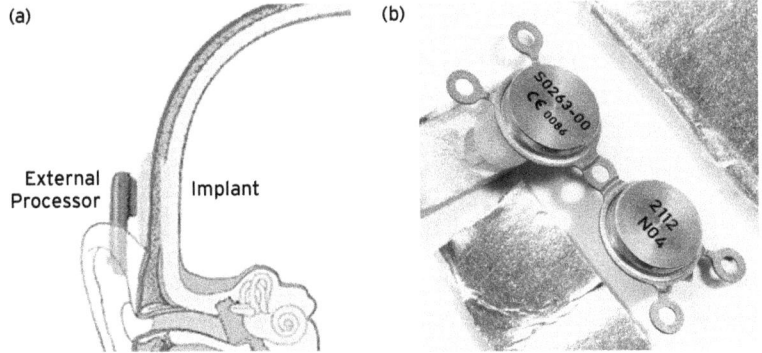

FIGURE 1-5 Sophono Bone Conduction System. (a) External processor converts sound and powers a flat magnet tightly adherent to the skull skin by a matching implant magnet (b) which is secured to bone by five 4 mm self-tapping microscrews. Sound vibrations are sent to the cochlea via bone conduction. Images courtesy of Sophono, INC.

Cochlear implant systems convert everyday sounds into coded electrical pulses. These electrical pulses stimulate the auditory nerve, and the brain interprets the pulses as sound (see diagram). The brain receives sound information within microseconds, so sounds are heard as they occur.

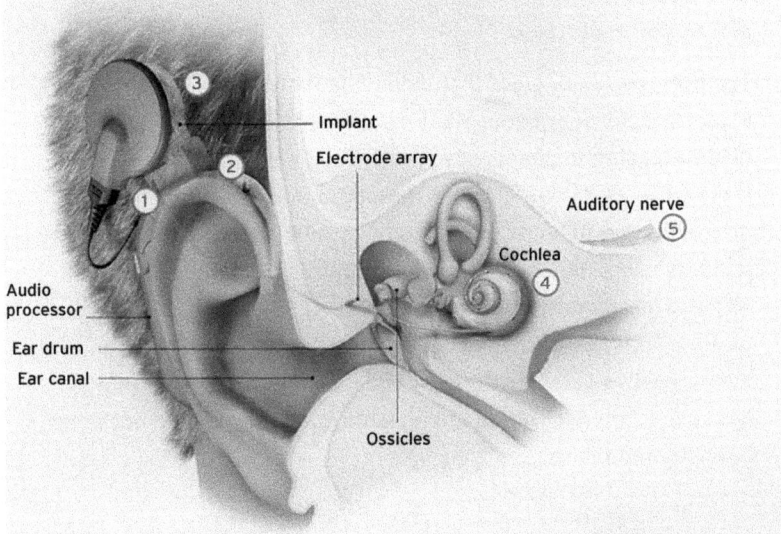

1. Sound is picked up by the microphone of the audio processor.
2. The audio processor analyzes and converts sounds into a special code.
3. This code is sent to the coil and transmitted across the skin to the implant.
4. The implant interprets the code and sends electrical pulses to the electrodes in the cochlea.
5. The auditory nerve picks up this signal and sends it to the auditory center in the brain. The brain recognizes these signals as sound.

FIGURE 1-6 Cochlear Implant System. Image courtesy of MED-EL Corporation, USA.

devices for implantation in the profound HL ear even if the contralateral audition is in the severe, not profound, range. These devices are surgically implanted and secured to the skull in a bony well in a 2-hour ambulatory procedure. They have electrode arrays that penetrate deeply into the cochlea resulting in a tonotropic electrical stimulation of the basilar membrane and auditory nerve (Figure 1-6). The procedure is highly successful with minimal risk factors (far less than risks associated with a simple tonsillectomy). Ideally bilateral implantation (simultaneous or sequential) offers better audition and localization of sound; however, often because of insurance coverage only one device is implanted. On average, cochlear implants have a lifetime 2% failure rate and may be successfully implanted and reimplanted starting at the age of 6 months, as long as the baby is 20 lbs or more. In the rare instances when there is congenital absence of the cochlea or cochlear nerve, an auditory brainstem implant may be successfully implanted on the cochlear nucleus; however, they do not provide nearly the same high-definition hearing as standard cochlear implants.[10,11]

> **KEY POINTS TO REMEMBER**
>
> - The average HL for older than age 55 is 9 dB per decade.
> - Most HL is sensorineural, bilateral, progressive with age, and loud noise exposure in genetically predisposed population.
> - If the HL is asymmetric with disproportionately poor speech discrimination patients may require an ABR or contrast brain/internal auditory canal (IAC) MRI to rule out a retrocochlear lesion and a work-up for auditory neuropathy.
> - All HL is amenable to rehabilitation techniques including hearing aids, assistive-listening devices, and on occasion surgery may help especially with implantable hearing processors and cochlear/brainstem implants.

Further Reading
1. Britton BH. Presbycusis. In: Anne S Patterson, editor. Common Problems in Otology. Mosby, St. Louis, MO 63146, 1991. pp. 281–91.

2. Fransen E, Lemkens N, Laer LV, et al. Age-related hearing loss impairment (ARHI): environmental meds factors and genetic prospects. Exp Gerontol 2003:38(4):353.
3. Lalwani AK. The aging inner ear. In: Anil K. Lalwani, editor. Current Diagnosis and Treatment in Otolaryngology-Head and Neck Surgery. Lange Medical Books/McGraw-Hill, New York, NY, 2004. pp. 735–42.
4. Berlin Cl, Hood L, Morlet T, et al. Auditory neuropathy/dys-synchrony: diagnosis and management. Mental Retard Dev Dis Res Rev 2003;9(4):225–31.
5. Frank RL. Hearing Loss in Older Adults: Who's Listening? JAMA. 2012;307(11):1147–8. doi:10.1001/jama.2012.321.
6. Breneman Al, Gifford RH, Dejong MD. Cochlear implantation in children with auditory neuropathy spectrum disorder: long term outcomes. J Am Acad Audiol 2012;23(1):5–17.
7. Kohan D, Levy L. Aural rehabilitation: hearing aids and assistive listening devices. SiPAC. Alexandria, VA: American Academy of Otolaryngology Head and Neck Surgery, 1999.
8. Cate M, Deguine O, Calmels MN, et al. BAHA or MedEl Vibrant Soundbridge: results and criteria of decision. Cochlear Implants Int 2011;12(Suppl. 1):S130–2.
9. Snik AF, Mylanus EA, Aroops DW, et al. Consensus statements on the Baha System: where do we stand at present? Am Otol Rhinol Laryngol Suppl 2005;195:2–12.
10. Budenz CL, Roland JT Jr, Babb J, et al. Effects of cochlear implant technology in sequentially bilaterally implanted adults. Otol Neurotol 2009;30(6):731–5.
11. Vincent C. Auditory brainstem implants: how do they work? Anat Rec (Hoboken) 2012;295(11):1981–6.

2 Sudden Sensorineural Hearing Loss

A 46-year-old white male flew home to New York City after a mandatory West Coast business trip. He had mild allergies or a respiratory infection and was sneezing frequently during the flight and felt nasal congestion with sinus and aural pressure, more on the left side. He had mild otalgia bilaterally on descent. A day later he woke up with severe left hearing loss (HL), static-like constant nonpulsatile noise in the ear, and increasing fullness. At presentation there is no ear pain, drainage, or dizziness. There is no history of prior ear disease. His past medical history is negative and he denies any medication intake. His neurologic and physical examinations are normal. The tuning fork tests and audiogram (Figure 2-1) reveal a severe left sensorineural HL (SNHL) and normal hearing on the right.

What do you do now?

Sudden HL (SHL) is defined as rapid onset of subjective hearing deterioration occurring within a 72-hour period in one or both ears. Conductive HL is very common and may be caused by cerumen impaction, infections, or lesions of the outer or middle ear and are not pertinent to this discussion because they are easily diagnosed and treated with ear canal cleaning and/or appropriate topical or systemic antibiotics.

The focus here is on sudden SNHL, which affects 5–20 per 100,000 of the population.[1] This condition is defined as a decrease greater than or equal to 30 dB, affecting at least three consecutive frequencies by comparison with preexisting recent audiogram or the opposite ear's threshold on a current test. The HL may involve the cochlea, auditory nerve, or higher aspects of central auditory perception or processing.

A total of 90% of SNHL is idiopathic at presentation and most likely secondary to viral, vascular, or autoimmune pathology.[2,3] Less common possible etiologies, such as Ménière's disease, central nervous system lesions, cerebrovascular accidents or ischemic events, and trauma are discussed later in this text.

Bilateral SHL may be caused by systemic infections (i.e., luetic otitis, Lyme disease) or central nervous system pathology. Metabolic disorders, such as renal disease, hyperviscosity, and ototoxic chemicals, may injure

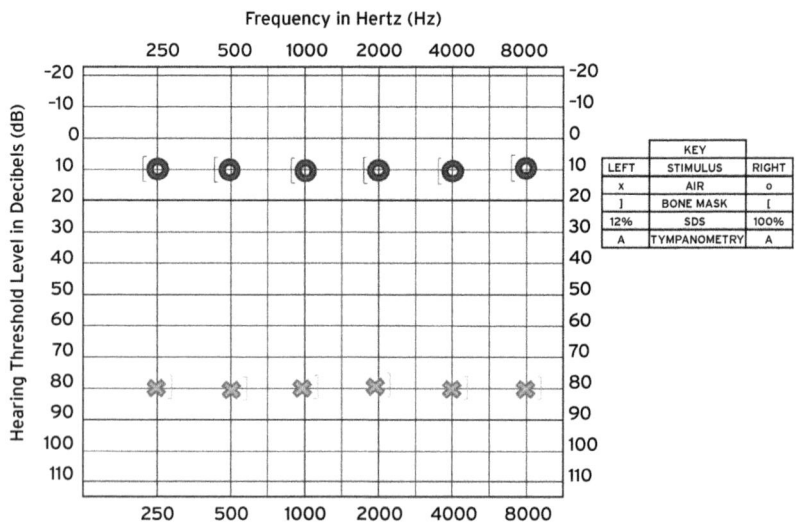

FIGURE 2-1 Audiogram reveals normal hearing on the right, and a severe/profound sensorineural hearing loss at all frequencies as well as poor speech discrimination score (SDS) on the left.

the cochlea. Progressive HL suggests the possibility of a perilymphatic fistula, labyrinthitis, or autoimmune disease.

At best about 60% of sudden SNHL (SSNHL) recovers spontaneously. Prognosis depends on the presentation, progression of the HL, configuration and severity of HL on the audiogram, the presence or absence of vertigo, the patient's overall health status, and how soon therapy is initiated postinjury. A younger healthier individual with a moderately to severe upsloping low-frequency HL has the best prognosis. Older medically challenged patients with more severe flat or downsloping audiograms, with poor speech discrimination, and vestibular symptoms have a far worse prognosis. Long-term follow-up and management is recommended because the etiology of the HL may eventually become evident, and progression of the hearing deficit may be prevented with targeted therapy.

HL and tinnitus frequently result in anxiety and depression, especially more significant in the elderly population, which may withdraw from interaction with society. The psychological adverse sequela of SSNHL must be properly addressed on a long-term basis in a comprehensive team approach including psychiatric consultation.[4,5]

The Academy of Otolaryngology has the following guidelines for managing SSNHL for patients 18 years or older. The protocol provides evidence-based recommendations and may be applied to our case presentation.[1]

1. Clinicians should distinguish SNHL from conductive HL in a patient presenting with SHL. The patient history and physical examination are most important in conjunction with tuning fork tests.
2. Clinicians should assess patients with presumptive SSNHL for bilateral deficits, recurrent episodes of HL, or focal neurologic findings. The physical examination and history are most important.
3. Clinicians should not order computed tomography of the head or brain on initial evaluation of a patient with presumed SSNHL unless there is a history of trauma.
4. Audiometry is required to diagnose presumptive idiopathic SSNHL. Confirmation is achieved if equal or greater than 30 dB HL is present at three consecutive frequencies versus contralateral

ear or preinjury audiogram. Lack of audiometry should not preclude initiation of treatment postdiscussion with the patient.

5. Clinicians should not obtain routine laboratory tests in the patient with idiopathic SSNHL. Targeted tests may be appropriate in some patients: Lyme titer in individuals living in endemic areas for this condition, Fluorescent Treponemal Antibody-absorption (FTA-Ab) titer for otosyphylis in high-risk population, autoimmune panel in patients highly suspected for this condition (i.e., someone with rheumatoid arthritis, lupus, and so forth).[6] Each patient work-up must be individualized.

6. Clinicians should evaluate patients with idiopathic SSNHL for retrocochlear pathology ideally with contrast-enhanced magnetic resonance imaging or alternatively with auditory brainstem response and subsequent audiometric follow-up.[7,8]

7. Clinicians should educate patients with idiopathic SSNHL about the natural history of the condition, benefits and risks of medical intervention, and the limitations of current acceptable treatment protocols.

8. Clinicians may offer corticosteroids as initial therapy to patients with idiopathic SSNHL. One common protocol is sequential or concomitant therapy with prednisone, 1 mg/kg twice daily with tapper every 3 days by 20 mg. The treatment usually is provided for 2 weeks. Intratympanic steroid perfusion usually consists of dexamethasone, 24 mg/cc, with 0.4 cc injected by a myringotomy weekly for about 3 weeks depending on patient response to therapy, and the side effects. The safety profile of steroids must be discussed with the patient in detail. Poorly controlled diabetes, immunocompromised status, tuberculosis, and peptic ulcerative disease are among the many conditions where the risks of systemic steroid applications are significant.[9-15]

9. Hyperbaric oxygen therapy offered within 3 months of diagnosis of idiopathic SSNHL may be helpful. This treatment option is controversial and not often available, even in major medical centers.[16,17]

10. Clinicians should not routinely prescribe antivirals, thrombolytics, vasodilator vasoactive substances, or antioxidants to patients with idiopathic SSNHL.

11. Clinicians should offer intratympanic steroid perfusion (same protocol as in point 8) when patients have incomplete recovery from idiopathic SSNHL after failure of initial management if this treatment has not already been used at initial presentation. This option is individualized based on what is considered by the patient and physician as a treatment "failure." Is a 50% improvement in the initial HL sufficient? Does the patient expect and desire even better results? Is the risk/benefit ratio favorable to the patient? These questions and answers remain in flux.[9-15]
12. Clinicians should obtain follow-up audiometric evaluations within 6 months of diagnosis of idiopathic SSNHL.
13. Clinicians should counsel patients with incomplete recovery of hearing about the possible benefits of amplification, hearing-assistive technology, and other supportive measures.[4]

In the case presented here the patient's aural fullness and discomfort is most likely caused by allergies and/or viral upper respiratory infections worsened by the barotrauma of the flight. A perilymphatic fistula is unlikely in a patient without trauma or any vestibular symptoms.

KEY POINTS TO REMEMBER

- Audiometry is required for diagnosis: 30-dB HL is present at three consecutive frequencies compared with contralateral ear or previous test.
- A total of 90% of SSNHL is idiopathic, most likely viral, noise-induced, vascular, or autoimmune etiology.
- A total of 60% of SSNHL recover spontaneously.
- The work-up should include a contrast brain/ Internal Auditory canal magnetic resonance imaging or auditory brainstem response study, and hematologic tests for Lyme, luetic otitis, or autoimmune disease.
- Initial therapy is started immediately not pending the diagnostic evaluation and includes high doses of systemic and intratympanic steroids, possibly hyperbaric oxygen therapy, but not antivirals.
- Long-term follow-up of audition is mandatory because deficit may progress.

Further Reading
1. Stahler RJ, Chandrasekhar SS, Archer SM, et al. AAO-HNS Clinical Practice Guideline. Sudden hearing loss. Otolaryngol Head Neck Surg 2012;146(3):S1-S35.
2. National Institute of Deafness and Communication Disorders. Sudden deafness 2000. Available from: http://www.NIDCD.NIH.GOV/health/hearing/suddenloss. Accessed May 18, 2011.
3. Rauch SD. Clinical practice: idiopathic sudden sensorineural hearing loss. N Engl J Med 2008;359(8):833–40.
4. Chisolm TH, Johnson CE, Danhauer JL, et al. A systematic review of health-related quality of life and hearing aids: final report of the AA of Audiology Task Force on the Health-Related Quality of Life Benefits of Amplification in Adults. J Am Acad Audiol 2007;18(2):151–83.
5. Chau JK, Len JR, Atashband S, et al. Systematic review of the evidence for the etiology of adult sudden sensorineural hearing loss. Laryngoscope 2010;120(5):1011–21.
6. Garcia Berrocal JR, Ramirez-Camacho R, Vargas JA, et al. Does the serological testing really play a role in the diagnosis of immune-mediated inner ear disease? ACTA Otolaryngol 2002;122(3):242–8.
7. Aarnisalo AA, Suoranta H, Ylikoski J. Magnetic resonance imaging findings in the auditory pathway of patients with sudden deafness. Otol Neurotol 2004;25(3):245–9.
8. Davidson HC. Imaging evaluation of sensorineural hearing loss. Semin Ultrasound CT MR 2001;22(3):229–49.
9. Rauch SD, Halpin CF, Antonelli PJ, et al. Oral vs. intratympanic corticosteroid therapy for idiopathic sudden sensorineural hearing loss: a randomized trial. JAMA 2011;305(20):2071–9.
10. McCall AA, Swan EE, Borenstein JT, et al. Drug delivery for treatment of inner ear disease: current state of knowledge. Ear Hear 2010;31(2):156–65.
11. Labus J, Breil J, Stulzer H, et al. Meta-analysis for the effect of medical therapy vs. placebo on recovery of idiopathic sudden hearing loss. Laryngoscope 2010;120(9):1863–71.
12. Jeyakumar A, Francis D, Doerr T, et al. Treatment of idiopathic sensorineural hearing loss. Acta Otolaryngol 2006;126(7):708–13.
13. Alexander TH, Weisman MH, Derebery JM, et al. Safety of high-dose corticosteroids for the treatment of autoimmune inner ear disease. Otol Neurotol 2009;30(4):443–8.
14. Filipo R, Covelli E, Balsamo G, et al. Intratympanic prednisone therapy for sudden sensorineural hearing loss: a new protocol. Acta Otolaryngol 2010;130(11):1209–13.
15. Seggas I, Koltsidopoulos P, Bibas A, et al. Intratympanic steroid therapy for sudden hearing loss: a review of the literature. Otol Neurotol 2011;32(1):29–35.

16. Gill AL, Bell CV. Hyperbaric oxygen: its uses, mechanism of action and outcomes. QJM 2004;97(7):385–95.
17. Bennett MH, Kertesz T, Young P. Hyperbaric oxygen for idiopathic sudden sensorineural hearing loss and tinnitus. Cochrane Database Syst Rev 2007;1:CD004739.

3 Noise-Induced Hearing Loss

A 49-year-old male, inner city high school gym teacher complains of increasing bilateral hearing loss (HL), far worse after chaperoning his teenage daughters at a loud concert 2 days earlier. He also has new severe bilateral whistling noises in his head keeping him up at night. His daughters also heard unusual mechanical noise in their head following the concert; however, the sounds disappeared in a few hours. He denies prior ear pathology. His local otolaryngologist noted a normal physical examination. The audiogram (Figure 3-1) revealed bilateral high-frequency moderate sensorineural hearing loss (SNHL) asymmetrically worse on the left at 4 kHz. He was told there is significant "nerve damage" and was offered amplification. The patient decided he needed a neurologic evaluation for his neural problem. Your physical examination and tuning fork tests are in agreement with his previous otolaryngologic evaluation.

What do you do now?

Noise-induced HL (NIHL) is very common and may be present in about 10 million U.S. citizens. Acoustic trauma louder than 85 dB either as an impulse or repeated exposure results in severe trauma to the organ of Corti in the cochlea. Initially the outer hair cells and later the inner hair cell stereocillia are damaged by the shearing forces of the tectorial membrane. This triggers a cascade of metabolic and vascular changes reducing electromotility resulting in a temporary HL (a temporary threshold shift), which may last for about 12 hours. With further loud noise exposure there is loss of stereocillia, vacuolization of the cell body, and later cell death, including the surrounding supporting cells (Hansen and Deiters). The stria vascularis degenerates and scar tissue replaces the dead cells resulting in a permanent threshold shift (PTS) with permanent SNHL. Following end-organ damage there is retrograde degeneration of the cochlear nerve.[1,2]

NIHL is more common in urban settings and affected by cultural parameters. Loud music exposure and the proliferation of portable audio devices have increased the risk of NIHL in the younger population.[3] Individual susceptibility to noise varies, and there is a definitive multifactorial genetic component. The outer ear sound transfer function peaks around 3–4 kHz, which corresponds to the peak NIHL noted at 4 kHz on audiograms. The severity of the NIHL correlates with both the duration and intensity of the

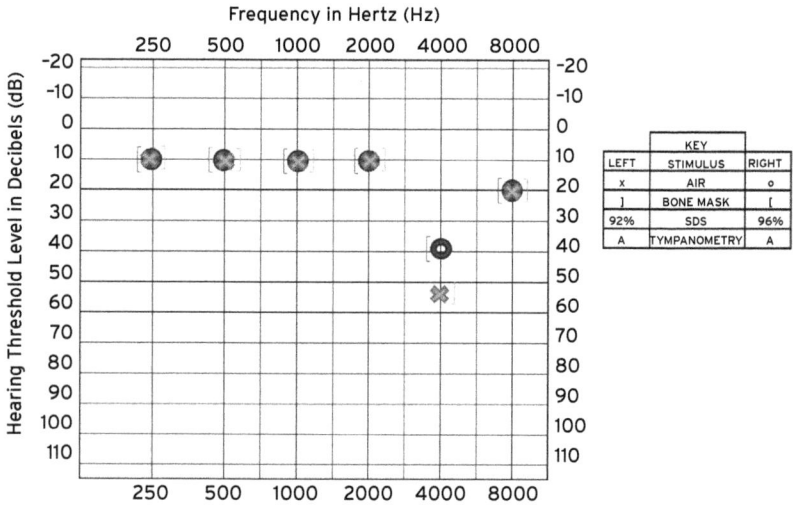

FIGURE 3-1 Audiogram reveals bilateral moderate sensorineural hearing loss with peak deficit at 4 K, asymmetrically worse on the left. There is bilateral normal speech discrimination.

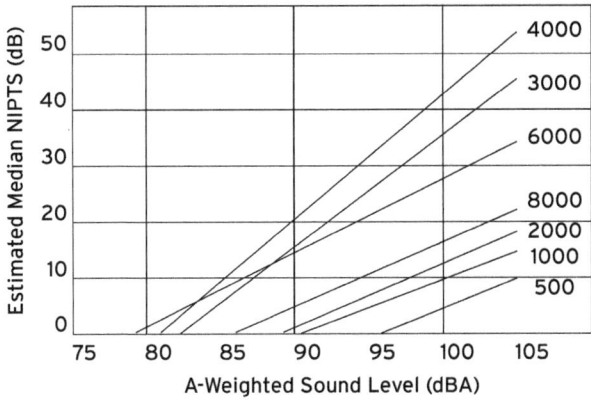

FIGURE 3-2 Estimated permanent threshold shifts at various frequencies produced by noise exposure of more than 10 years duration. (Source: Lalwani AK. Occupational hearing loss. In: Anil K. Lalwani, editor. Current Diagnosis and Treatment in Otolaryngology-Head & Neck Surgery. Lange Medical Books/McGraw-Hill, New York, NY, 2004. p. 783.)

offending sounds (Figure 3-2). The high-frequency range of the cochlea is most susceptible to chronic loud noise exposure. Speech discrimination is preserved until the deficits move laterally on the frequency scale from the 4 kHz peak to the lower frequencies of the speech range.[1,4]

The acoustic reflex in the middle ear with contracture of the stapedius and tensor tympani muscles stiffens the conductive mechanism for noises above 90 dB. However, there is a delay of about 100 milliseconds in the activation of this protective mechanism, which helps attenuate continuous loud noise but provides no benefit for high-intensity impulse noise (i.e., explosions), which is thus more damaging. Efferent olivocochlear projections from the brainstem to the outer hair cells activated by loud noise hyperpolarize these cells reducing the electromotility response and the cochlear amplifier, thus providing another layer of protection from damaging loud sounds.

Tinnitus almost always accompanies acoustic trauma. The severity of the HL does not necessarily correlate to the intensity and frequency of occurrence, or the frequency spectrum of tinnitus. NIHL does not progress after the noxious noise is removed. The Occupational Safety and Health Administration in 1983 defined requirements for hearing conservation in noisy work environments. For unprotected ears the allowed exposure time decreases by one-half each 5-dB increase in the average noise level starting at 85 dB (Table 3-1).[4,5] The Occupational Safety and

TABLE 3-1 **Permissible Noise Exposure in the Workplace**

Hours Per Day	Sound Levels dBA (Slow Response)
16	85
8	90
6	92
4	95
2	100
1	105
0.5	110
0.25	115

Source: Lalwani AK. Occupational hearing loss. In: Anil K. Lalwani, editor. Current Diagnosis and Treatment in Otolaryngology-Head & Neck Surgery. Lange Medical Books/McGraw-Hill, New York, NY, 2004. p. 784.

Health Administration mandated that 8 hours or more exposure to 85 dB or greater (time-weighted average) at a workplace triggers implementation of a hearing-conservation protocol. The program includes the following:

1. Noise monitoring: frequency, intensity, and duration of the offending noise are constantly monitored.
2. Engineering controls: develop ways to isolate the source of noise (enclosures, barriers, distance) from susceptible individuals.
3. Administrative controls: determine ways to diminish noise intensity and exposure at work.
4. Worker education: proper training must be provided for employees and management to understand the risks of noise exposure, with retraining on an annual basis.
5. Hearing protection devices: mandatory when noise averages more than 90 dB during an 8-hour day. Ear plugs (premolded or custom made), canal caps, and ear muffs all reduce noise by 15–30 dB if continuously used and properly fitted. They effectively block the ear canal or the ear with an airtight seal. The ear plugs are better for low-frequency noise protection,

whereas the ear muffs are better for dampening high-frequency noise. Simultaneous use of both appliances adds 10–15 dB more protection than when used alone, and should be used in combination for exposure to noise levels 105 dB or greater. Normal-hearing individuals wearing noise protection devices should still be able to understand a regular conversation even in a quiet setting.

6. Audiometric evaluation: to be performed on a routine basis and the data freely provided to workers and management.

The only treatment available for PTS-NIHL is amplification, assistive-listening devices, and noise reduction or avoidance in the future. The criteria for amplification are similar to those discussed previously in the chapter on presbycusis.[4,5]

Tinnitus therapy includes multivitamins (usually include variable amounts of niacin, lipoflavonoid, vitamin C, *Ginko biloba*, and so forth), tinnitus masking techniques, biofeedback therapy to suppress tinnitus, and occasionally psychiatric consultation for associated anxiety and/or depression.[6-9]

Comorbidities may lead to progressive HL and tinnitus (i.e., presbycusis; metabolic diseases, such as diabetes mellitus or renal disease; autoimmune disorders). Ingestion of ototoxic substances (i.e., cisplatinum, quinine) may enhance patient susceptibility to noise trauma.

When a patient presents with sudden SNHL (SSNHL) or tinnitus following noise exposure, the injury may be a temporary threshold shift. Although controversial, such patients may respond to rapidly provided high doses of systemic or intratympanic steroids with a similar protocol as frequently offered to other patients with SSNHL unrelated to noise.[10,11]

In the case presentation, the middle-age patient's work exposure to loud noise in the school environment was exacerbated by the loud concert he attended 48 hours earlier. The HL in this case represents a PTS. He may still benefit from steroid therapy. A work-up to differentiate the diagnosis is mandatory even though the etiology in this case seems obvious. Preexisting pathology is often only diagnosed when there is a sudden change that brings the patient's attention to the newly perceived deficit.

> **KEY POINTS TO REMEMBER**
> - Acoustic trauma more than 85 dB and repeated exposure injures the organ of Corti especially at the basal turn of the cochlea resulting in high-frequency auditory deficits.
> - Patient education on how to preserve and protect audition is mandatory.
> - Auditory rehabilitation should be offered if the deficit is more than mild.

Further Reading

1. Jackler RK, Brackmann DE. Neurotology, 2nd edition. Mosby, Philadelphia, Pennsylvania 19106, 2005.
2. Le Press CG, Yamashita D, Minami SB, et al. Mechanism of noise-induced hearing loss indicates multiple methods of prevention. Hear Res 2007;226(12):22–43.
3. Gilles A, De Ridder D, Van Hal G, et al. Prevalence of leisure noise-induced tinnitus and the attitude towards noise in university students. Otol Neurotol 2012;33(6):899–906.
4. Lalwani AK. Occupational hearing loss. In: Anil K. Lalwani, editor. Current Diagnosis and Treatment in Otolaryngology-Head & Neck Surgery. Lange Medical Books/McGraw-Hill, New York, NY, 2004. pp. 781–92.
5. Suter AH. The gearing conservation amendment: 25 years later. Noise Health 2009;11(42):2–7.
6. Hobson J, Chisholm E, El Reface A. Sound therapy (masking) in the management of tinnitus in adults. Cochrane Database Syst Rev 2012;11:CD006371.
7. Baldo P, Doree C, Molin P, et al. Antidepressants for patients with tinnitus. Cochrane Database Syst Rev 2012;9:CD003853.
8. Salvi R, Lobarinas E, Sun W. Pharmacological treatments for tinnitus: new and old. Drugs Future 2009;34(5):381–400.
9. Enrico P, Sirca D, Mereu M. Antioxidants, minerals, vitamins, and herbal remedies in tinnitus therapy. Prog Brain Res 2007;166:323–30.
10. Tabuchi K, Murashita H, Sakai S. Therapeutic time window of methylprednisolone in acoustic injury. Otol Neurotol 2006;27(8):1176–9.
11. El-Hennawi DM, El-Deen MH, Abou-Halawa AS, et al. Efficacy of intratympanic methylprednisolone acetate in treatment of drill-induced sensorineural hearing loss in guinea pigs. J Laryngol Otol 2005;119(1):2–7.

4 Ototoxins

A 35-year-old mildly obese male with known sleep apnea and restless leg syndrome has been on therapy for 3 months with quinine and a continuous positive airway pressure device. His symptoms of snoring, daytime fatigue, and nightly leg movements have improved. In an attempt to lose weight he has been exercising and swimming every day. He presents to the emergency room with 1 week of increasingly severe diffuse headaches, episodes of blurry vision, nausea with vomiting, ringing in the ears, aural fullness with muffled hearing, and nonpositional fluctuating dizziness and vertigo. His past medical history is unremarkable, he is afebrile, and the physical examination is only significant for mild ataxia. The tuning fork tests are inconclusive, the head computed tomography ordered by the emergency room is normal, and his audiogram reveals a high-frequency moderately severe asymmetric hearing loss (HL), worse on the right (Figure 4-1). The speech discrimination score (SDS) is bilaterally normal, as are his tympanograms.

What do you do now?

Ototoxicity is a result of functional impairment and cell degeneration of the cochlea and eighth cranial nerve caused by toxic effects of certain therapeutic agents. In contrast, neurotoxicity involves damage at higher levels of processing within the brainstem and central auditory and vestibular pathways, which also involves audition and balance. Most commonly used compounds that are ototoxic and vestibulotoxic are aminoglycoside and macrolide antibiotics; loop diuretics; antineoplastic agents, such as cisplatinum; salicylates; quinine; and less frequently exposure to heavy metals (Table 4-1).[1] Ototoxicity is usually potentiated by loud noise exposure, preexisting sensorineural HL, concomitant or sequential exposure to multiple ototoxic substances, and diminished hepatorenal function.[1,2] Most adverse sequelae of exposure to ototoxic medications are reversible. Monitoring for otovestibular toxicity involves serial otoacoustic emission, audiograms (especially high-frequency testing), and electronystagmography. The history and physical examination are still the best modalities for evaluating what is clinically pertinent otovestibular pathology.

Keeping patients well hydrated, monitoring renal and hepatic function, controlling the plasma drug concentration, nonbolus distribution of compounds, and judicious limited use of otovestibulotoxic drugs provides the best strategy for prevention of adverse side effects. Hypothetic

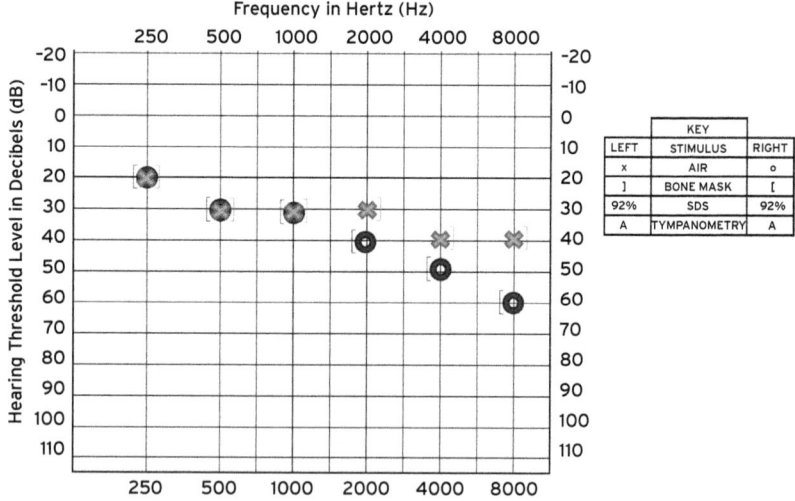

FIGURE 4-1 Audiogram reveals asymmetric right high frequency severe sensorineural hearing loss versus a moderate deficit on the left. There is bilateral normal speech discrimination.

TABLE 4-1 **Ototoxic Drugs**

Aminoglycoside antibiotics

    Streptomycin

    Dihdrostreptomycin

    Kanamycin

    Gentamicin

    Neomycin

    Amikacin

    Tobramycin

    Netilmicin

Vancomycin

Erythromycin

Chemotherapeutic agents

    Cisplatin

    Nitrogen mustard

Loop diuretics

    Furosemide

    Ethacrynic acid

Salicylates

Quinine

Source: Hughes GB, Pensak ML. Clinical Otology, 2nd edition. New York: Theime, 1997. p. 163.

coadministration of iron chelators and free radical scavengers with careful monitoring of plasma concentration of toxic substances in patients with renal and hepatic pathology may reduce the otovestibulotoxic effects.[2,3]

Aminoglycosides are effective bactericidal antibiotics used for gram-negative and enterococcal infections with inhibition of protein synthesis by ribosomes. Otovestibular toxicity occurs in up to 16% of patients receiving therapeutic dosages with the side effects distributed equally between cochlear and vestibular function. Toxicity may occur well after the antibiotic regimen is completed. Cochleotoxicity is more severe with kanamycin, neomycin, and amikacin. Vestibulotoxicity is greater with streptomycin, tobramycin, and gentamycin. Basal outer hair cells and Type I cells (especially in the utricle) are more susceptible to damage by free radicals. With progression of damage the rest of the otic capsule is affected with retrograde degeneration of ganglions and neurons. Initial calcium antagonism and channel blockade is reversible only early during antibiotic therapy. HL higher than 25 dB, delayed onset, immediate onset with progression despite discontinuation of drug, and continued drug use despite evidence of toxicity are all associated with irreversible injury. Aminoglycoside nephrotoxicity is usually reversible, but not otovestibular toxicity. Initial HL is usually high frequency, but progresses with increased duration of antibiotic therapy. The injury may be unilateral or bilateral and asymmetric. Toxicity is related to the total amount of antibiotic given, not the inner ear fluids or plasma concentration (which correlates better to nephrotoxicity). Previous exposure to ototoxic drugs, hyperthermia, dehydration, and bacteremia potentiate toxicity of aminoglycosides. Most patients with documented otovestibulotoxicity are asymptomatic. There is a strong genetic predisposition to aminoglycoside otovestibulotoxicity. Genetic mutations in maternal ribosomal and mitochondrial RNA may explain up to one-third of familial cases. Impaired hepatorenal status, loud noise exposure, and neonatal status aggravate toxicity.[2-5]

Loop diuretics, such as furosemide and ethacrynic acid, inhibit oxidative phosphorylation and succinic dehydrogenase action producing a reversible dose-related decrease in endocochlear potentials with increase in sodium and decrease in potassium concentration in endolymph with loss of ionic transport. The most severe damage is noted at the stria vascularis, although cochlear basal hair cells and Type I and II cells also degenerate. Most often the HL is reversible within 2–3 days. Continued use of high dose of loop diuretics may result in permanent deficits.[6]

Acetylsalicylic acid, a metabolite of aspirin, is well known to result in reversible sensorineural HL, tinnitus, and rarely vertigo by blocking outer hair cell electromotility diminishing the cochlear amplifier. The HL is usually moderate, dose-related, and reversible within a few weeks of cessation of therapy.[7]

Quinine and its derivatives are used for leg cramps at night, malaria therapy, and arrhythmias. These cinchona tree alkaloids affect mostly the stria vascularis, although degeneration of the organ of Corti, especially at the basal turn, has been documented. The case presented in this chapter demonstrates cinchonism, or quinine toxicity, which presents with cochleovestibular symptoms, gastrointestinal upset, and occasionally blurry vision. Only symptomatic therapy is warranted because quinine toxicity is almost always self-limiting and reversible. An appropriate work-up of the patient presented would include a contrast brain magnetic resonance imaging to rule out a central nervous system lesion. Cessation of quinine therapy with rapid resolution of symptoms confirms the diagnosis.[2,7,8]

Macrolide antibiotics, such as erythromycin and clarithromycin, inhibit protein synthesis at the ribosomes and are effective in infections by B-hemolytic streptococci, *Streptococcus pneumoniae*, staphylococci, and *Legionella*. A flat moderate HL, tinnitus, and vertigo usually occur only at high doses and there is usually rapid recovery within a day of stopping the antibiotics.[2,9]

Antineoplastic agents, such as cisplatin, may be life-saving and are frequently used despite the numerous nephrotoxic and otovestibulotoxic side effects associated with therapy. The tinnitus and HL is usually high frequency, irreversible, and cumulative dose related. Vestibular side effects are less frequent and less severe. Pathology is attributed to iron-induced free radicals, which injure the organ of Corti at the basal turn of the cochlea. Concurrent therapy with fosfomycins may prevent the toxic effects on the otic capsule. Increased hydration and diuresis may prevent renal toxicity but not ototoxicity.[10,11]

Numerous other agents may be ototoxic to varying degrees. Most commonly encountered are caffeine, nonsteroidal anti-inflammatory medications, nicotine, alcohol, industrial solvents, iodine, and some metals. Careful monitoring of cochlear and vestibular function may determine when ototoxic medication should be withdrawn or alternatives used.[2,9,11]

KEY POINTS TO REMEMBER

- Most common ototoxic and vestibulotoxic medications are aminoglycoside and macrolide antibiotics, loop diuretics, antineoplastic agents, salicylates, quinine, and heavy metals.
- Most ototoxicity is reversible.
- Monitoring renal and hepatic function and control of plasma drug concentration is key to prevention.
- HL is sensorineural preferentially involving the outer hair cells of the basal turn of the cochlea thus affecting the high frequencies.

Further Reading
1. Hughes GB, Pensak ML. Clinical Otology, 2nd edition. New York: Theime, 1997. p. 163.
2. Jackler RK, Brackmann DE. Neurotology, 2nd edition. Elsevier Mosby, Philadelphia, Pennsylvania 19106, 2005. pp. 593–5.
3. Tabuchi K, Nishimura B, Nakamagoe M, et al. Ototoxicity: mechanism of cochlear impairment and its prevention. Curr Med Chem 2011;18(31):4866–71.
4. Selimoglu E. Aminoglycoside-induced ototoxicity. Curr Pharm Des 2007;13(1):119–26.
5. Bates DE. Aminiglycoside ototoxicity. Drugs Today (Barc) 2003;39(4):277–85.
6. Ikeda K, Oshima T, Hidaka H, et al. Molecular and clinical implications of loop diuretic ototoxicity. Hear Res 1997;107(1–2):1–8.
7. Jang TT, Rhee CK, Lee CS, et al. Ototoxicity of salicylate, nonsteroidal anti-inflammatory drugs, and quinine. Otolarybgol Clin North Am 1993;26(5):791–810.
8. Tange RA, Dreschler WA, Claessen FA, et al. Ototoxic reactions of quinine in healthy persons and patients with *Plasmodium falciparum* infection. Auris Nasus Larynx 1997;24(2):131–6.
9. Norris CH. Drugs affecting the inner ear: a review of their chemical efficacy, mechanism of action, toxicity, and place in therapy. Drugs 1988;36(6):754–72.
10. Hyppalto MA, De Oliveira JA, Rossato M. Cisplatin ototoxicity and otoprotection with sodium salicylate. Eur Arch Otorhinolaryngol 2006;263(9):798–803.
11. Yorgason JG, Fayad JN, Kalinec F. Understanding drug ototoxicity: molecular insights for prevention and clinical management. Expert Opin Drug Saf 2006;5(3):383–99.

5 Congenital Hearing Loss

A 1-year-old boy adopted at birth in the United States presents with newly diagnosed bilateral profound sensorineural hearing loss (SNHL). According to the adoptive parents the biologic parents were reported as healthy, with normal hearing, and the gestation and delivery were uneventful. The child is meeting developmental milestones except babbling is diminished, and the parents believe the child is not responding to their voice. The pediatrician reports the child's physical examination was normal. He was sent for pediatric audiologic evaluation where the otoacoustic emissions and auditory brainstem response tests reveal a profound bilateral SNHL. A cochlear implant was recommended. The parents worry about other "nerve damage" and want an expert's advice on possible other neurologic deficits.

What do you do now?

Congenital HL is the most common of sensory deficits at birth. Permanent moderate-to-severe SNHL prevalence at birth is believed to be 1–3 per 1000 live births. Many more children have other conditions, such as atresia, stenosis, or meconium in narrow ear canals resulting in conductive HL. Here we focus on the neural deficits that may involve neurologists. Maternal infections, such as rubella and meningitis, perinatal ototoxic environmental exposure, trauma, and newborn cytomegalovirus infections may result in HL. However, genetic hereditary HL (HHL) is far more common. There may be up to 400 genes involved in HL. A total of 70% of HHL is nonsyndromic with the remaining 30% syndromic. Autosomal-recessive transmission accounts for about 80% of nonsyndromic HL (designated DFNB), whereas the remaining 18% is mostly autosomal-dominant (designated DFNA). A small percentage (1%–2%) of HHL may be caused by mitochondrial maternal transmission and X-linked heredity (DFN) (Table 5-1).[1-4]

Nonsyndromic HHL usually involves three genes that encode connexin, pendrin, and myosins. These proteins are involved in ion homeostasis, cytoskeleton hair cell structures including motility, cell-to-cell interaction, and transcription. Connexins are involved in homeostasis and are transmembrane proteins that form channels for intercellular transport resulting in recycling potassium ions back into the endolymph post hair cell activation, thus maintaining appropriate potentials for the next auditory

TABLE 5.1 **Relative Incidence of Inheritance Patterns in Hereditary Hearing Impairments**

Mode of Inheritance	Percent
Autosomal recessive	60%–70%
Autosomal dominant	20%–25%
X-linked recessive	2%–3%
Chromosomal	<1%
Mitochrondrial	<1%
Multifactorial	Not known

Source: Hughs GB, Pensak ML. Clinical Otology, 2nd edition. New York: Thieme, 1997. p. 270.

stimulus. Gap Junction Beta 2 (connexin 26) gene deletion is the most common cause of recessive profound SNHL (about 50% of these patients). Two single base pair deletions (35delG and 167delT) represent half of the mutations in this gene.[2,5]

Pendrin is a polypeptide involved in renal, thyroid, and cochlear metabolism including sulfur transport and iodide and chloride ions. Mutations involving SLC26A4 (PDS) pendrin formation may result in 10% of HHL and isolated large vestibular aqueduct, the most common radiologic anomaly involving congenital deafness. In patients with large vestibular aqueduct during life up to 40% progress to profound HL with minor trauma. The parents of these children are counseled on how to protect their children and minimize risk of head injury.[6]

Myosins are actin-dependent molecular engines needed for proper function of mechanosensory hair cells. They are also involved in stabilizing the basal attachments of stereocilia in regulating ion channels, and movement of vesicles within the hair cell cytoplasm. Mutations in myosis have been linked to multiple nonsyndromic HHL.[1-3]

Syndromic HHL involves multiple other clinical and anatomic abnormalities besides the HL. Most syndromes are autosomal-dominant. Table 5-2 provides a summary of most frequent syndromes, their clinical findings, gene locus involved, and target organ.[3]

In the case presented in this chapter the child is adopted, and the family history provided was incomplete but negative for HL or syndromes. A very thorough history and physical examination is mandatory to rule out abnormalities associated with syndromic HL, such as preauricle pits and pigmentation abnormalities. The auditory work-up was already completed with otoacoustic emissions and auditory brainstem response tests confirming the severity of HL. A multidisciplinary approach involving the pediatrician, geneticist, otolaryngologist, audiologist, speech pathologist, ophthalmologist, cardiologist, and neurologist is mandatory for treating these patients, especially if a syndrome is suspected. Urine analysis, thyroid function test, electrocardiogram, temporal bone computed tomography and/or brain magnetic resonance imaging (fast-spin echo T2-weighted images or contrast-enhanced scans) may be necessary. A genetic screen may be appropriate for adequate counseling of the family. Auditory rehabilitation is initiated as soon as possible and may involve amplification,

TABLE 5.2 **Syndromic Hereditary Hearing Impairment: Clinical Findings Besides Hearing Loss and Associated Genes**

Syndrome	Clinical Findings	Gene		
		Name	Function	Localization
Pendred syndrome (AR)	Goiter; most common syndrome; deafness about 10% congenital bilateral moderate-to-severe sloping	PDS	Anion transporter?	Endolymphatic duct sack utricle, saccule, cochlea; enlarged vestibular aqueduct and Mondini defect possible
Waardenburg syndrome (AD)	Dystopia canthorum; pigmentary abnormalities of hair, iris, and skin; 2%–5% congenital HL; up to 50% deaf; abnormal vestibular function	MITF, PAX3, SOX10	Transcription factors	Neural crest–derived cells
		EDN3, EDNRB	Cell development	Melanoblast, neuroblast precursors
Usher syndrome (AR)	Retinitis pigmentosa; 8% of congenital deafness; many types depend on presence or lack of vestibular pathology; most common syndrome to affect eyes and ears	MYO7A	Cell maintenance?	Hair cells
		USH1C	Protein-protein interaction?	Organ of Corti, saccule, utricle
		CDH23	Cell organizer?	Inner, outer hair cell
		PCDH15	Development of hair cells?	Sensory epithelium, inner ear
		USH2A	Development/ homeostasis?	Basement membrane
		USH3		Various tissues
Alport syndrome (X-linked dominant)	Renal dysfunction (hematuria with progressive renal failure); ocular abnormalities (lenticonus and retinal flecks); 1% of congenital HL; high-frequency SNHL	COL4A3, COL4A4, COL4A5	Collagen formations	Outer sulcus, inne sulcus, basilar membrane, spiral ligament of cochlea

TABLE 5.2 **(Continued)**

Syndrome	Clinical Findings	Gene		
		Name	Function	Localization
Branchio-oto-renal syndrome (AD)	Branchial derived anomalies (cleft, cysts, or fitulas); otologic anomalies (pits, HL); 2% congenital HL; renal malformations	EYA1, other genes?	Role in development of inner ear?	Vestibular organ, inner ear
Neurofibromatosis type II (AD)	Bilateral vestibular schwannomas, meningiomas, schwannomas, gliomas, neurofibromas in the scalp; juvenile subcapsular cataract; symptoms in late childhood	NF2 gene	Tumor suppressor gene	Schwannoma cells
Jervell and Lange-Nielsen syndrome (AR)	Prolonged QT interval with syncopal attacks and possible death; 0.25% congenital SNHL	KVLQT1, KCNE1	Potassium channel	Stria vascularis
Treacher Collins syndrome (AD)	Hearing loss caused by malformations in the middle and inner ear; craniofacial abnormalities (mandibulofacial dysostosis)	TCOF1	Nucleolarcytoplasmic transport?	Neural folds, branchial arches
Stickler syndrome (AD)	Conductive hearing loss possible; eye findings (high myopia, cataract); arthropathy (spondyloepiphyseal dysplasia); cleft palate	COL2A1, COL11A1, COL11A2	Collagen protein	Tectorial membrane

AD = autosomal dominant; AR = Autosomal recessive.
Adapted from: Lalwani AK. Current Diagnosis & Treatment in Otolaryngology-Head & Neck Surgery. Hereditary Hearing Impairment. Lange Medical Books/McGraw-Hill, New York, NY, 2004. p. 746.

assistive-listening devices, bone-anchored hearing processors, cochlear implants, and a proper educational environment.[5,7,8] Cognitive deficits are not frequent in this setting, but developmental delay may occur because of poor audition. Some patients may be referred to neurology for vestibular symptoms associated with syndromic and nonsyndromic HHL.

> **KEY POINTS TO REMEMBER**
>
> - Congenital HL is the most common sensory deficit at birth.
> - 70% of HHL is nonsyndromic.
> - Autosomal-recessive transmission accounts for 80% of nonsyndromic hearing deficits.
> - Connexin 26 gene deletion is the most common cause of recessive profound bilateral SNHL.
> - A multidisciplinary team approach is required for diagnosis, monitoring deficits, and to provide rehabilitation.

Further Reading
1. Hughes GB, Pensak ML. Clinical Otology, 2nd edition. New York: Thieme, 1997.
2. Jackler RK, Brackmann DE. Neurotology, 2nd edition. Elsevier Mosby, Philadelphia, Pennsylvania 19106, 2005.
3. Lalwani AK. Current Diagnosis & Treatment in Otolaryngology-Head & Neck Surgery. Hereditary Hearing Impairment. Lange Medical Books/McGraw-Hill, New York, NY, 2004.
4. Korver AM, Admiraal RJ, Kant SG, et al. Causes of permanent childhood hearing impairment. Laryngoscope 2011;121(2):409–16.
5. Kohan D, Sorin A, Hanin L. Evaluation and Rehabilitation of the Hearing-Impaired Child SiPac-2ndEd. Am Acad Otolaryngol-Head Neck Surg Foundation, Alexandria, VA, 2006.
6. Mori T, Westerberg BD, Atashband S, et al. Natural history of hearing loss in children with enlarged vestibular aqueduct syndrome. J Otolaryngol Head Neck Surg 2008;37(1):112–8.
7. Beswick R, Driscoll C, Kei J. Monitoring for postnatal hearing loss using risk factors: a systematic literature review. Ear Hear 2012;33(6):745–56.
8. Kohan D, Levy L. Aural Rehabilitation: Hearing Aids and Assistive Listening Devices; SiPac-American Academy of Otolaryngology-Head and Neck Surgery Foundation, Alexandria, VA, 1999.

6 Neurofibromatosis

A 16-year-old white female grade A student presents with increasing headaches for 6 months. One year ago she noticed progressive left hearing loss (HL), fullness, and nonpulsatile tinnitus, which became constant a few months ago. The right ear is normal. There is no other pertinent otolaryngologic history. Her father, who was adopted, and had a severe unilateral HL died in a motor vehicle accident at age 28, when the patient was 2 years old. She wears glasses since age 12. The rest of her past medical history, family history, social history, and review of systems is unremarkable. The microscopic otologic examination is normal. Neurologic evaluation is unremarkable. She has two café-au-lait macules larger than 15 mm. The tuning fork tests indicate left nonconductive HL. Her audiogram (Figure 6-1) reveals a left profound sensorineural HL and poor discrimination.

What do you do now?

This case presents us with a seemingly healthy young woman with unilateral severe progressive sensorineural HL and tinnitus, headaches, and long history of impaired vision. The family history is limited by the early accidental death of her father. There is no history of recent trauma, viral infection, or loud noise exposure. She was sent for a brain magnetic resonance imaging (MRI) (Figure 6-2) where a large left

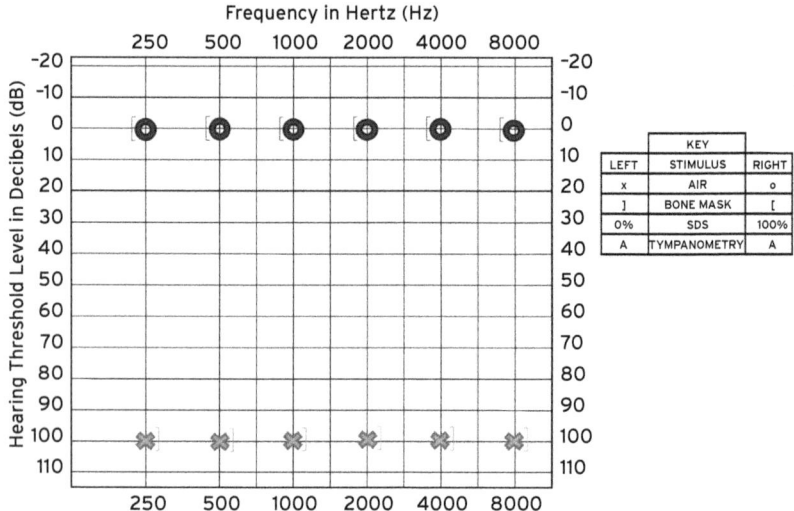

FIGURE 6-1 Audiogram reveals asymmetric left profound sensorineural hearing loss with 0% speech discrimination, and normal hearing on the right.

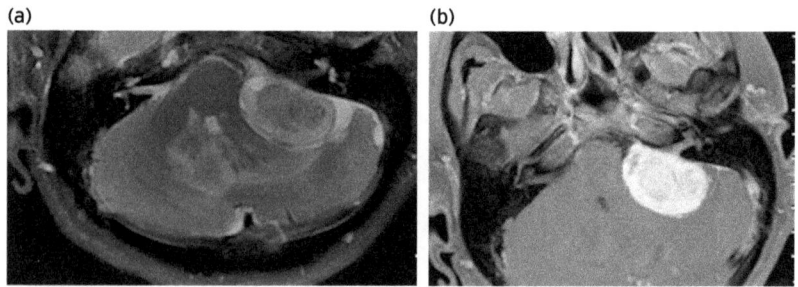

FIGURE 6-2 Contrast enhanced Brain MRI demonstrating a large left acoustic schwannoma with cerebellar and 4th ventricle compression. (a) axial FIESTA view, (b) axial T1 with Gadolineum view. (Source: private collection of Dr. Roy Holliday, Chairman of Head and Neck/Neuroradiology, New York Eye and Ear Infirmary, New York, NY).

cerebellopontine angle lesion consistent with an acoustic neuroma is evident. She underwent an ophthalmologic evaluation, which revealed posterior subcapsular lenticular opacities. Further questioning of the mother reveals that she always thought the child's father may have had a HL, but he died so young suddenly thus it was never evaluated. Considering the patient's diagnosis and presentation, the father's hearing deficit may also have been from an Internal Auditory Canal or cerebellopontine angle lesion. The diagnosis is most likely neurofibromatosis 2 (NF2), or central NF.[1,2]

NF2 is distinguished from NF1, or Recklinghausen disease/peripheral NF, by both molecular genetics and clinical presentation. The incidence of NF2 is 10 times less than for NF1, at 1:30,000 to 1:50,000. In 50% of patients with NF2 there is a new germline mutation with the remainder having autosomal-dominant inheritance. There is almost 100% gene penetrance but various expressivity. Most patients present in the second or third decade of life. The NF2 gene is located on chromosome 22, whereas the NF1 gene is on the long arm of chromosome 17. Merlin, the NF2 gene, is involved in tumor suppression and growth regulation. This lack of suppression results in early tumor formation.[1-5]

NF1 is defined as having two or more of the following:

- Six or more café-au-lait macules; >5 mm prepuberty or >15 mm postpuberty
- Two or more neurofibromas or plexiform neurofibromas
- Freckling in axillary or inguinal areas
- Optic glioma
- Two or more iris hamartomas (Lisch nodules)
- An osseous lesion, such as thinning of the long bone cortex or sphenoid dysplasia
- A first-degree relative with NF1

NF2 diagnostic criteria for definitive pathology are as follows:

- Bilateral vestibular schwannomas (VS) (Figure 6-3) or family history of NF2 (first-degree relative) plus:
  - Unilateral VS <30 years old or
  - Any two of meningioma, glioma, schwannoma, juvenile posterior subcapsular lenticular opacities, or
  - Cortical cataracts

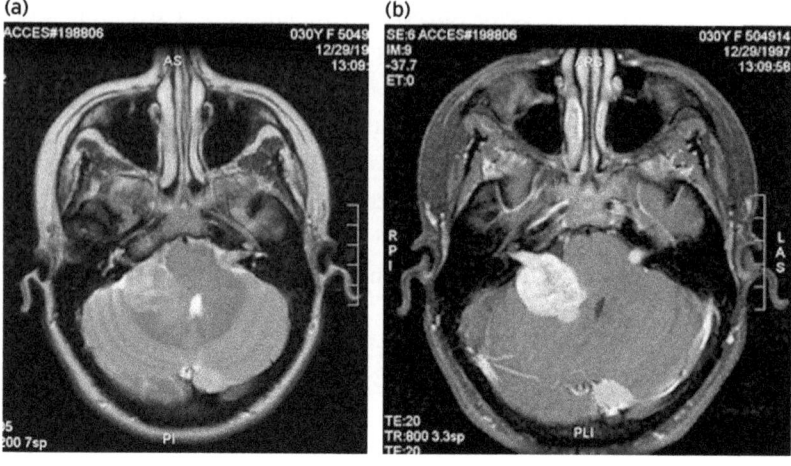

FIGURE 6-3 Neurofibromatosis Type 2. Axial T2 MRI demonstrating bilateral acoustic schwannomas, right much larger than the left. A small meningioma is present left of midline in the cerebellum. (a) axial T2, (b) Axial T1FS with Gadolineum. (Source: private collection of Dr. Roy Holliday, Chairman of Head and Neck/Neuroradiology, New York Eye and Ear Infirmary, New York, NY).

NF2 diagnostic criteria for probable pathology are:

- Unilateral VS <30 years old plus at least one of meningioma, glioma, schwannoma, juvenile subcapsular lenticular opacities, or cataracts
- Multiple meningiomas (two or more) plus unilateral VS <30 years of age or one of following: meningioma, glioma, schwannoma, juvenile subcapsular lenticular opacities, or cataracts

A proper work-up for NF2 should include a contrast-enhanced MRI of the brain and spine, and audiologic and ophthalmologic evaluation. Genetic testing of the patient and frequently the family is appropriate for adequate counseling. The MRI scans are repeated annually for continuous monitoring.[5,6] Prognosis for NF2 depends on clinical severity and gene expressivity. Overall neoplasms associated with this condition are more aggressive than sporadic tumors. They are more infiltrative of surrounding neurovascular structures and complete tumor removal with preservation of function of surrounding neural anatomy is almost impossible.

Stereotactic radiosurgery and multiple tumor decompression procedures play a dominant role in management. Therapy is discussed in greater detail in the Acoustic Schwannoma chapter of this text. Genetic counseling is a very important component in managing NF2. A team approach involving numerous specialties is best in optimizing treatment and rehabilitation of the myriad of clinical deficits associated with NF2.[7-10]

KEY POINTS TO REMEMBER

- NF1 and NF2 are distinguished by both genetics and clinical presentation; please learn the listed definitions for each entity.
- The diagnostic evaluation and monitoring requires brain and spine contrast-enhanced MRI performed annually, and genetic testing and counseling of the patient and family.
- Stereotactic radiosurgery and multiple tumor decompression are the mainstays of therapy in a multidisciplinary approach to tumor control and rehabilitation.

Further Reading

1. Yohay K. Neurofibromatosis types 1 and 2. Neurologist 2006;12(2):86–93.
2. Ferner RE. Neurofibromatosis 1 and neurofibromatosis 2: a twenty-first century perspective. Lancet Neurol 2007;6(4):340–51.
3. McClatchey AL. Neurofibromas. Annu Rev Pathol 2007;2:191–216.
4. Hoa M, Slattery WH III. Neurofibromatosis 2. Otolaryngol Clin North Am 2012;45(2):315–32.
5. Rodriguez D, Young Poussaint T. Neuroimaging findings in neurofibromatosis Type 1 and 2. Neuroimaging Clin N Am 2004;14(2):149–70.
6. Jackler KJ, Brackmann DE. Neurotology, 2nd edition. Elsevier/Mosby, Philadelphia, Pennsylvania 19106, 2005. pp. 783–91.
7. Parsons CM, Canter RJ, Khatri VP. Surgical management of neurofibromatosis. Surg Oncol Clin N Am 2009;18(1):175–96.
8. Szudek J, Briggs R, Leung R. Surgery for neurofibromatosis 2. Curr Opin Otolaryngol Head Neck Surg 2012;20(5):347–52.
9. Colletti L, Shannon R, Colletti V. Auditory brainstem implants for neurofibromatosis type 2. Curr Opin Otolaryngol Head Neck Surg 2012;20(5):353–7.
10. Tysome JR, Macfarlane R, Durie-Gair J, et al. Surgical management of vestibular schwannomas and hearing rehabilitation in neurofibromatosis type 2. Otol Neurotol 2012;33(3):466–72.

7 Vestibular Schwannomas and Menigiomas

A 60-year-old male, corporate executive has mild progressive hearing loss for a few years. He listened to loud music in his youth. In the boardroom he requires bilateral hearing aids for the last 5 years. Six months ago he noticed the right ear was getting worse and now he had constant nonpulsatile tinnitus at night. He has relatively new mild disequilibrium without vertigo. He denies other otologic symptoms but had minor head trauma with a motor vehicle accident 6 years ago. The head computed tomography (CT) at the time was normal. The past medical history is negative. His parents had hearing loss with ageing. His internist recommends a neurologic evaluation. The full physical examination is normal. The tuning fork test is inconclusive because he has a bilateral hearing loss.

What do you do now?

First we look at the new audiogram and compare with the old one revealing a significant decrease in right audition over a relatively short time period (Figure 7-1). Next, he needs a brain/internal auditory canal (IAC) magnetic resonance imaging (MRI) (Figure 7-2). The diagnosis is now clear: a 2 cm acoustic neuroma (AN). ANs (more correctly schwannomas) represent 6%–8% of intracranial tumors and are the most common lesions at the cerebellopontine angle (CPA). A total of 95% are sporadic with mean presentation at 50 years of age, whereas the remaining 5% are noted with neurofibromatosis (NF) type 2 and present earlier in life, mean age 31 years old. These schwannomas arise from the vestibular division of the eighth cranial nerve with equal origin from the superior and inferior components. There are two histologic patterns: Antoni A, densely packed cells with small spindle-shaped dense nuclei; and Antoni B, loose cellular aggregates of vacuolated pleomorphic cells found in larger tumors. There is no difference in associated clinicopathology between the two types and both have microinvasion of surrounding nerve fibers and compression resulting in symptoms. There is rare malignant degeneration. The tumors typically begin in the IAC and grow slowly, unless there are cystic areas with intratumor hemorrhage resulting in a much more rapid expansion of the lesion.

Usual symptoms are asymmetric slow progression of unilateral hearing loss, tinnitus, and vertigo with small IAC tumors. Later, with penetration into the cistern (CPA), the hearing loss and tinnitus progress; however, vertigo resolves and is replaced by disequilibrium. With eventual brainstem compression headaches, ataxia, hypesthesia of trigeminal nerve, and facial and lower cranial nerve deficits occur. Compression of the fourth ventricle results in hydrocephalus and associated severe neurologic symptoms.[1,2] Tumor growth is 1–3 mm per year, and up to 30% show no growth, whereas 22% grow more than 2 mm per year. The mean growth rate for all AN was 1.8 mm per year; however, among the 54% of tumors demonstrating radiographic growth the mean growth rate jumped to 4 mm per year.[3] Tumor measurements are based on the CPA three-axis component with additional mention of extent of IAC involvement and total tumor volume.

Diagnostic tests include audiometry. There is usually an asymmetric sensorineural hearing loss with disproportionate decrease in speech discrimination. The auditory brainstem response is abnormal in about 85%–90% of patients with AN greater than 1 cm in size. However, the false-positive

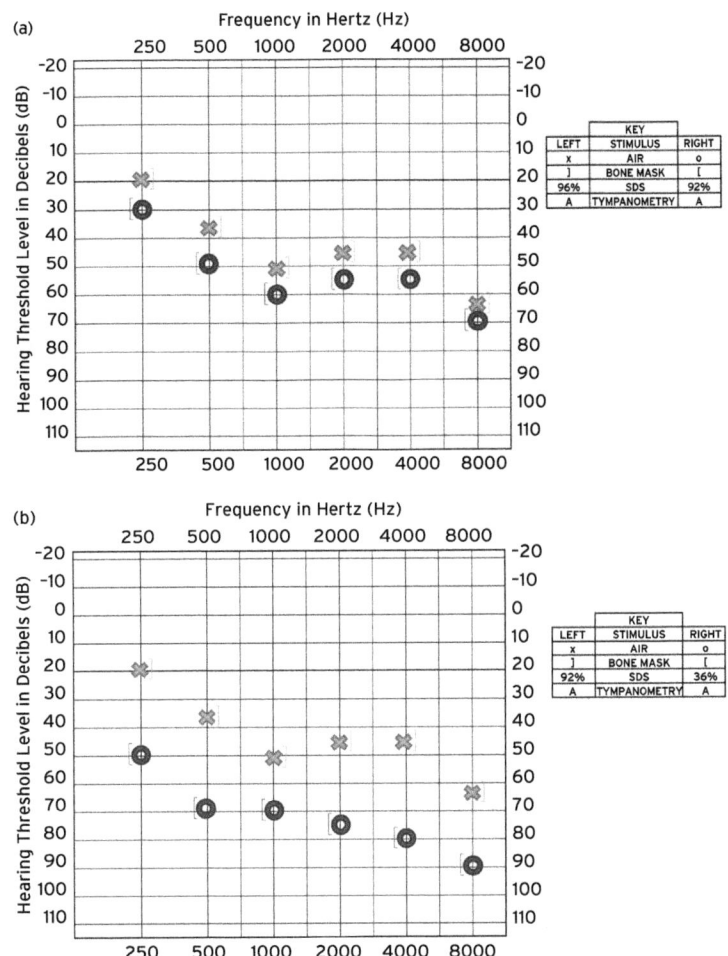

FIGURE 7-1 (a) Audiogram from 2008 showing bilateral moderately severe sensorineural hearing loss, with a mild asymmetry worse on the right, but bilateral normal speech discrimination. (b) Six months later the audiogram on the same patient shows asymmetric progression of now severe slopping to profound right sensorineural hearing loss with disproportionate decrease in speech discrimination.

rate is about 80%. Stacked auditory brainstem response is a more accurate technique gaining in popularity. The caloric response in electronystagmography tests the superior vestibular nerve (the lateral semicircular canal) and is abnormal in 98% of AN originating from this nerve. Inferior vestibular nerve lesions, if large enough to compress the IAC blood supply or the

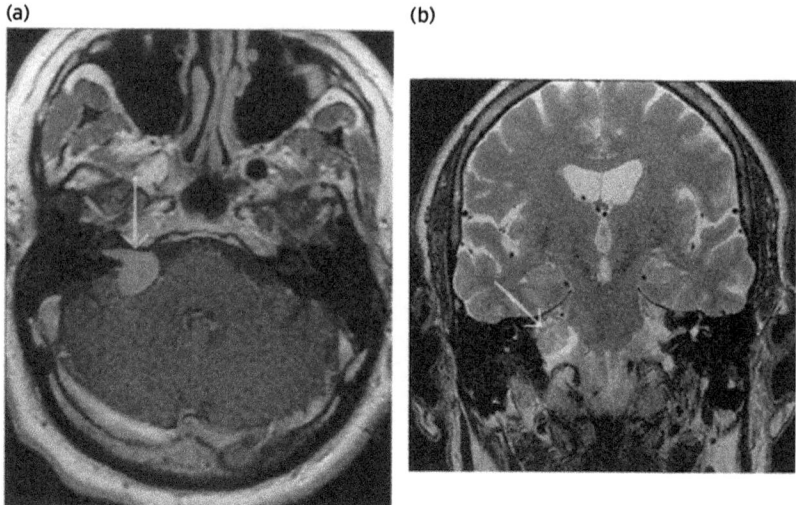

FIGURE 7-2 (a) Axial contrast enhanced T1 MRI of brain reveals a two cm right acoustic schwannoma. (b) Coronal T2 brain MRI of the same patient. (Source: author personal collection.)

superior vestibular nerve, also have abnormal electronystagmography in up to 50% of patients. Contrast-enhanced MRI is the gold standard for diagnosing AN, with a 98% accuracy and specificity for lesions 3 mm or larger.[3,4] For claustrophobic patients open MRIs are almost as accurate. Contrast-enhanced CT scans are slightly less accurate and are used in patients with contraindications for MRI.

Patients with small tumors, the elderly, individuals in poor health or with minimal symptoms, or those with documented slow-growing tumors may decide on conservative management, observation, with regular audiologic and radiologic studies at 6- to 12-month intervals.[5]

Stereotactic irradiation (SI) by the Gamma Knife (Cobalt 60) or a single source linear accelerator (Cyber Knife) induce tumor necrosis in irradiated lesions by a large dose delivered in a single session or a few fractions over a very short time period. Proton beams may be more effective than the photon-beam radiation that is more popular today. These techniques minimize radiation exposure to adjacent tissues. The treatment delivers about 25 Gy to the tumor center and 12–14 Gy to the margin. Because of inflammation the tumor usually swells the first 6–18 months; however, the lesions shrink in about two-thirds of patients over a longer time period. Regrowth occurs in about 5% of AN, a higher rate for cystic lesions. Hearing is preserved in up to 60% of patients over about 5 years; however, the trend is for further severe loss of residual audition if follow-up is longer. Facial and trigeminal nerve irritative complications occur 6–12 months post therapy in approximately 5% if the tumor margin dose is limited to 12 Gy. The rate of complications is much higher if the dose at the tumor periphery is above 12–14 Gy.[2,6] Malignant degeneration following SI has been reported and hypothetically projected to be 1% at 10 years, 2% at 20 years, and 3% at 30 years post therapy.[7] Radiosurgery is reserved for tumors 4 cm or smaller in older individuals or those with complicated medical histories and documented tumor growth. If this modality fails to control the tumor, then the surgical options are still available. However, microsurgery in a radiated field is technically more difficult with a higher complication rate.[8-10]

Surgery is generally performed in younger patients with growing tumors and progressive symptoms. The technique varies with tumor size, location, and cranial nerve deficits. Tumors of any size with poor hearing (speech discrimination 50% or less) or tumors 2.5 cm or larger regardless of hearing acuity may be removed by the translabyrintine technique. Small tumors in the IAC just penetrating the CPA with good hearing may be removed by the middle fossa (MF) technique. Acoustic neuromas 1.5 cm or larger with good hearing may be excised by the retrosigmoid (RS) approach. The MF technique is most challenging with the narrowest field of vision, but gives the best exposure for distal lesions in the IAC in patients with salvageable hearing.[1,2,9] Total tumor excision is desirable and achieved in about 90% of cases. However, near total excision, where the residual lesion is a thin capsule less than 2 mm thick or residual tumor volume less than 25 mm square may be performed to spare key neurovascular structures. If the tumor remnant is distally in the IAC or at the brainstem where there is good vascular supply, the recurrence rate is higher than at other locations with impaired blood supply. Tumors with near total excision have a recurrence rate of 3% versus subtotal excision where the rate is 30% if more than 25 mm square of tumor mass was left behind.[11] Cauterization of tumor residual reduces incidence of regrowth.[1,2] Some neurosurgeons opt to decompress tumors for symptom relief and to avoid damaging key neurovascular structures than complete therapy with SI. Tumor follow-up is with contrast-enhanced MRI and fat-saturated technique at 3 years for total excision, and annual for incomplete tumor removal for the first 5 years, then biannual if no growth was detected.

Surgical mortality is less than 1% and is caused by ischemia; postoperative hemorrhage; meningitis; or air embolism, which usually occur in large tumors. The overall complication rate of surgery is 20%. Anteroinferior cerebellar artery injury is rare and results in ataxia and dysmetria, which slowly improve with therapy.[12] Cerebrospinal fluid (CSF) leak is the most common serious complication occurring in 5%–15% of patients. Usually it presents as otorhinorrhea, rarely as wound seepage. The incidence is not related to tumor size or approach. Treatment involves diuretics (e.g., Diamox), stool softener, bed rest, and lumbar subarachnoid drain for 3–5 days, and is 85% effective. Oversawing the incision in translabyrintine usually eliminates wound seepage. Subtotal petrosectomy with closure of external ear canal and eustachian tube is used as a last resort with almost 100% rate of cure of CSF leaks. Meningitis occurs in 2%–10% of patients and is usually associated with CSF leaks, and peaks 3.5 days postoperative. Limited perioperative use of antibiotics has decreased the incidence of meningitis. Antibiotics are of course appropriate once infection is documented with a spinal tap. Therapy is initiated before culture results. Aseptic meningitis caused by meningeal inflammation secondary to blood products and bone dust peaks 5 days postoperative and responds to corticosteroids and anti-inflammatory agents. Facial nerve injury may occur because of direct trauma during tumor dissection, thermal injury, or damage to the vascular supply. The anatomic integrity of the facial nerve is maintained in up to 97% of patients, yet at 1 year postoperative 20% of patients have mild to moderate paresis (grade 2–3 on House/Brackmann scale) and up to 4% have complete paralysis. Most paresis resolves within 2 months, but for more severe injury hyperfunction with twitching is common. Botox may help limit the facial tics. Intraoperative facial nerve monitoring and cortical bulbar stimulation and monitoring help prevent nerve injury during dissection. Delayed facial nerve paresis is caused by edema or reactivation of dormant herpes virus; the prognosis is excellent when patients receive corticosteroids and antivirals. If facial nerve injury is noted at surgery, primary anastomosis end-to-end or with cable graft (i.e., sural or greater auricular nerves) is performed at primary procedure. Later reconstruction may be performed with facial to hypoglossal anastomosis or cross facial nerve anastomosis with good results (usually grade 3 House/Brackmann function) noted around 16 months postsurgery. Eye protection to prevent corneal injury may require gold weight implants in the upper eye lid and/or tarsorrhaphy.[1,2]

Hearing loss is frequent regardless of the surgical technique. With MF measurable hearing is achieved in about 50% of patients, but useful hearing is only 25%. With RS surgery useful hearing is also only attained in 25% of patients, only on "favorable" tumors. Long-term outcomes are even worse with slow deterioration of audition most likely caused by restricted blood flow and increased fibrous scarring even when the tumor is totally resected. Rehabilitation involves standard amplification and devices that use bone conduction to transmit sound from the affected ear to the contralateral "normal" ear by bone-anchored hearing processors, Sophono, or the SoundBite system as discussed in chapter 1. Tinnitus is a common relatively minor complication and occurs in 50% of postsurgical patients. The incidence and severity is higher if the cochlear nerve is spared at surgery. Vestibular dysfunction is frequent and responds to vestibular therapy. Headaches are very common and mild the first year after surgery. The incidence is highest in RS patients presumably because of bone dust in the CPA. Nonsteroidal anti-inflammatory therapy and steroids help.

The patient presented here decided on observation and audiologic tests and MRI at 6-month intervals. Further therapy depends on rate of tumor growth, symptoms, and patient preference.

Meningiomas are the most common intracranial neoplasms accounting for about 20% of lesions; however, they are second to acoustic neuromas at the CPA. Most are benign and asymptomatic. They represent up to 30% of incidental tumors found at autopsy.[1,2,13] The peak incidence is the sixth and seventh decade of life. There is a female to male 3:2 ratio implying that female sex hormones may promote tumor growth. When present in children they are more aggressive. Meningiomas are the most common radiation-induced neoplasm of the central nervous system. A total of 95% of meningiomas are sporadic and about 2% hereditary, usually in NF2, which is autosomal-dominant with a propensity to develop multiple meningiomas and schwannomas. A total of 35% of patients with NF2 have meningiomas. Merlin is a protein functioning in tumor suppression and its formation is impaired by a mutation on the long arm of chromosome 22 as noted in patients with NF2.

Meningiomas are derived from arachnoid cap cells, the external layer of the arachnoid membrane. They have a broad firm attachment to dura. A total of 25% of lesions are hyperostotic and have calcified psammoma bodies.[2,4] The lesions are always highly vascular. There are three types:

Classical: Grade I lesion, representing 90% of meningiomas

Atypical: Grade II lesion, about 7%; on average four mitosis per high power field; they have a high recurrence rate after excision

Anaplastic: Grade III lesions, about 3%; on average 20 mitosis per high power field; even with aggressive intervention they have a poor prognosis (Table 7-1)

Meningiomas have a variable presentation when in the CPA and the audiovestibular test results do not correlate to tumor size.[13,14] CT and MRI reveal a well-circumscribed extra-axial mass, sessile with broad dural attachment. There is contrast enhancement on CT and T1-weighted MRIs (Figure 7-3). The T2-weighted MRI is heterogeneous. A total of 15%–20% of tumors have calcifications noted on CT and more than 50% reveal peritumor edema. MRI can detect lesions as small as 3 mm.[2-4]

Treatment is based on symptomatology and tumor aggressiveness and involves both surgical excision often preceded by embolization to diminish vascularity and/or radiosurgery. Complete excision is frequently impossible and subtotal excision is often performed. Slow tumor growth may be monitored radiologically.

TABLE 7-1 **World Health Organization Histopathologic Classification for Meningiomas**

World Health Organization Grade	Incidence	Histologic Subtype	Recurrence/ Aggressiveness
Grade I–Typical	Common	Meningothelial, fibrous, transitional, psammomatous, angiomatous	Low
	Rare	Secretory, microcystic, lymphoplasmacyte-rich, metaplastic	Low
Grade II–Atypical		Atypical, clear-cell, chordoid	Low
Grade III–Anaplastic		Anaplastic, papillary, rhabdoid	High
		Tumors with high proliferation index or brain invasion	

Source: Louis DN, Scheithauer BW, Budka H, et al. Meningiomas. In: Kleithues P, Cavenee WK, editors. Pathology and Genetics of Tumors of the Nervous System. Lyon: IARC Press, 2000. p. 314.

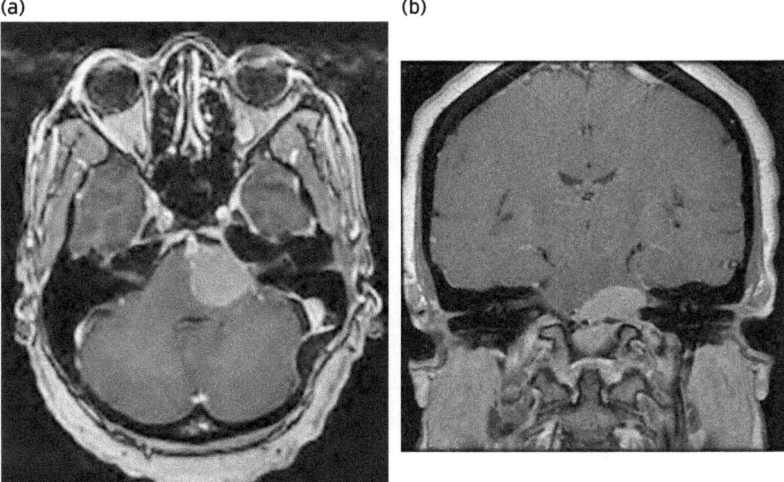

FIGURE 7-3 Large left meningioma without internal auditory canal (IAC) penetration, axial (a) and coronal (b) T1 contrast enhanced brain MRI. (Source: private collection of Dr. Roy Holliday, Chairman of Head and Neck/Neuroradiology, New York Eye and Ear Infirmary, New York, NY).

KEY POINTS TO REMEMBER

- The most common tumors of the CPA are almost always benign, overwhelmingly acoustic schwannoma (AN) and meningiomas, with epidermoids far less frequent but just as pathologic.
- Most patients present with asymmetric slowly progressive unilateral hearing loss; tinnitus; disequilibrium; and much later with facial nerve, trigeminal nerve, lower cranial nerves, and compressive symptoms.
- Tumor growth is on average 1–3 mm per year, whereas 30% show no growth.
- The evaluation includes audiometry and contrast-enhanced brain/IAC MRI.
- Tumor size, symptom complex, and patient medical status determine treatment options, which include observation, radiosurgery, or surgical excision of lesion (total or decompression).

Further Reading

1. Ho SY, Kveton JF. Acoustic neuroma. Assessment and management. Otolaryngol Clin North Am 2002;35(2):393–404.
2. Jackler RK, Brackmann DE. Neurotology, 2nd edition. Elsevier/Mosby, Philadelphia, Pennsylvania 19106, 2005.
3. Selesnick SH, Johnson G. Radiologic surveillance of acoustic neuromas. Am J Otol 1998;19:846–9.
4. Harnsberger HR, Wiggins III RH, Swartz JD, et al. Temporal bone: top 100 diagnoses. Amirys/W.B. Saunders, Philadelphia, Pennsylvania/Salt Lake City, Utah, 2003.
5. Raut W, Walsh RM, Bath AF, et al. Conservative management of vestibular schwannomas: a second review of a prospective longitudinal study. Clin Otolaryngol Allied Sci 2004;29(5):505–14.
6. Flickingger JC, Kondziolka D, Niranjan A, et al. Results of acoustic neuroma radiosurgery: AN analysis of 5 years experience using current methods. J Neurosurgery 2001;94:1–6.
7. Erfuth EM, Bulow B, Mikoczy Z, et al. Is there an increase in second brain tumors after surgery and irradiation for pituitary tumors? Clin Endocrinol (Oxf) 2001;55:613–6.
8. Schulder M, Sreepada GS, Kwartler JA, et al. Microsurgical removal of vestibular schwannoma after stereotactic radiosurgery: surgical and pathologic findings. Am J Otol 1999;20:364–7.
9. Pollock BE, Lunsford LD, Kondziolka D, et al. Vestibular schwannoma management. Part II. Failed radiosurgery and the role of delayed microsurgery. J Neurosurgery 1998;89:949–55.
10. Limb CJ, Long DM, Niparko JK. Acoustic neuromas after failed radiation therapy: challenges of surgical salvage. Laryngoscope 2003;115(1):93–9.
11. Bloch D, Oghalai JS, Jackler RK, et al. The role of less-than-complete resection of acoustic neuroma. Otolaryngol Head Neck Surg 2004;130:104–12.
12. Lee H, Kim JS, Chung EJ, et al. Infarction in the territory of anterior inferior cerebellar artery: a spectrum of audiovestibular loss. Stroke 2009;40(12):3745–51.
13. Kane PJ, Sughrue ME, Rutkowski MJ, et al. Clinical and surgical considerations for cerebellopontine angle meningiomas. J Clin Neurosci 2011;18(6):755–9.
14. Matsui T. Therapeutic strategy and long-term outcome of meningiomas located in the posterior cranial fossa. Neurol Med Chir (Tokyo) 2012;52(10):704–13.

8 Rare Tumors of the Cerebellopontine Angle

A 38-year-old male, elementary school principal, complains of childhood ear infections, worse on the right, requiring multiple surgeries. He developed a cholesteatoma, and at age 12 underwent a tympanomastoidectomy with tumor removal resulting in a severe right hearing loss but a dry healthy-appearing ear. He was stable until the last 6 months when he noticed increasing right aural pressure, facial tics, and occasional facial pain. His dental evaluation was normal. He has become mildly unsteady with exercise but has no other otologic symptoms. He denies head trauma and the past medical history is unremarkable. The physical examination is normal other than mild lower facial tics, which he attributes to job-related stress. The tuning fork tests are consistent with right hearing loss. An audiogram performed at school revealed a profound asymmetric right sensorineural hearing loss with very poor discrimination. The school nurse and visiting pediatrician are worried about his facial tics and recommend a neurologic evaluation.

What do you do now?

One should start by getting the correct imaging study: a brain/internal auditory canal (IAC) contrast magnetic resonance image (MRI) (Figure 8-1). A large mass is noted in the right cerebellopontine angle (CPA) consistent with an epidermoid, most likely from an incompletely excised cholesteatoma in his childhood. In another patient a temporal bone computed tomography (CT) (Figure 8-2) reveals a large destructive lesion of the petrous apex with

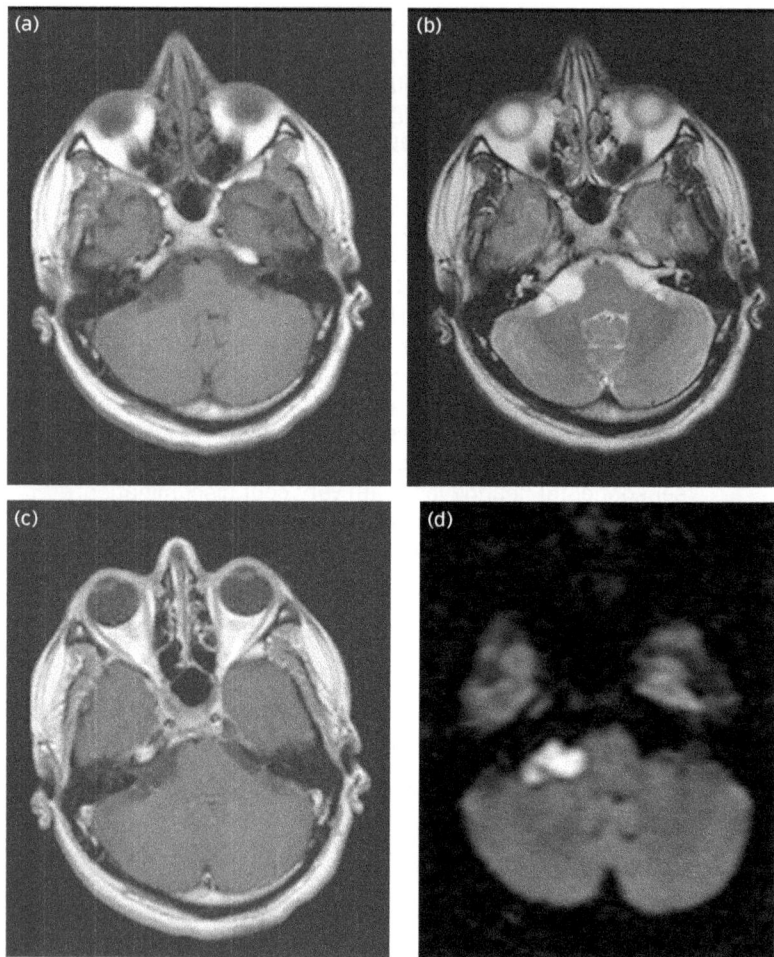

FIGURE 8-1 T2 brain MRI. Axial T1 (a), axial T2 (b), axial T1 with contrast (c), and axial diffusion weighted images (d) of right cerebellopontine angle epidermoid with minimal internal auditory canal penetration. (Courtesy of private collection of Dr. Roy Holliday, Chairman of Head and Neck/Neuroradiology, New York Infirmary, New York, NY.)

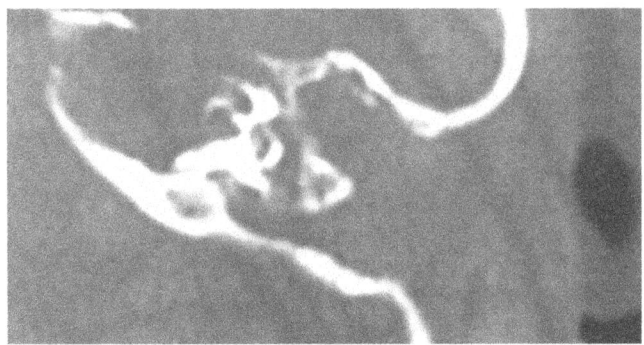

FIGURE 8-2 Temporal bone noncontrast computed tomography showing epidermoid with severe destruction of otic capsule, petrous apex, and central nervous system penetration.

severe bone erosion consistent with an acquired cholesteatoma or a congenital epidermoid. The lesion may penetrate the IAC and possibly the CPA.

The most common CPA tumors are vestibular schwannomas (acoustic neuromas) and meningiomas. The third most common lesion in this area is epidermoids, as presented in this case. Epidermoids represent up to 1.5% of all intracranial tumors, with the posterior fossa as the most common location. They originate from epithelial cell rests of the first branchial groove, consist of stratified squamous epithelium over a thin layer of connective tissue, and contain keratin debris and cholesterol crystals. In the case presented here the lesion was acquired and grew into the petrous apex, IAC, and possibly into the CPA. The tumors grow by migration along the planes of least resistance frequently enveloping key neurovascular structures. When cystic, they may spill content causing local inflammation. They are most frequently identified in the third and fourth decade of life after extensive tumor growth. On presentation 80% of patients have asymmetric hearing loss and tinnitus, 20% have disequilibrium and headaches. Facial tic douloureux and spasms may occur in up to 20%.[1] Temporal bone CT reveals a homogenous nonenhancing low-density mass with bone erosion. On MRI the mass has a low T1 signal, nonenhancing with contrast, and a high T2 signal. Fluid attenuated inversion recovery MRI signal is high because of protein content, in contrast to arachnoid cyst in the same location, which is hypointense. Diffusion sequence MRI has the same presentation as the fluid attenuated inversion recovery images.[2-5]

Treatment is surgical excision by a retrosigmoid, translabyrinthine, middle fossa, or transcochlear approach and depends on hearing level, cranial nerve involvement, extent of tumor, and if lesion crossed the midline to the contralateral side. Complete removal is attempted without cranial nerve sacrifice. There is a high morbidity associated with total tumor removal, and because there is slow tumor growth, subtotal excision is frequent with up to 30% patients requiring reoperations in the distant future. Aseptic meningitis and chronic inflammation may predispose malignant transformation of these lesions into squamous cell carcinoma with rapidly progressive symptoms and very poor prognosis.[1,6,7] The patient presented here opted to wait and have serial CT scans at 6-month intervals. He is young and understands surgery is unavoidable; however, he wanted to determine tumor growth rate and postpone the procedure for as long as safely possible.

Other rare lesions of the CPA are noted in Table 8-1.[1] Inflammatory and autoimmune lesions including sarcoidosis, Lyme disease, tertiary syphilis, aspergillosis, tuberculosis, and cysticerosis may rarely present with CPA syndrome. We focus next on relatively more common pathology at the CPA requiring intervention.

Intracranial lipomas are congenital, of mesodermal origin, and slow growing. Most are supratentorial and in the corpus callosum. They present with fluctuating hearing loss, tinnitus, and dizziness. Hemifacial spasms are relatively frequent. On CT the lesions are hypointense, but are hyperintense on T1 and T2 MRI consistent with fat. On T1 contrast fat signal fades. Surgery consists of decompression if symptoms progress. However, total tumor removal is unlikely because lipomas infiltrate surrounding nerve fibers, and sacrifice of the nerves should be avoided.[7,8]

Arachnoid cysts represent up to 10% of CPA lesions, are congenital, and usually asymptomatic and benign. If large they may obstruct causing hydrocephalus and CPA-associated symptoms. MRI and CT are diagnostic, and surgical drainage and shunting is rarely required.[1,9]

Primary brain neoplasms of the CPA represent 0.3% of lesions at this site. They present with rapid progression of symptoms when compared with acoustic neuromas and meningiomas. There is frequent intracranial hypertension and papilledema. Gliomas, astrocytomas, and oligodendrogliomas arise from the lateral medullary vellum of the lateral recess of the fourth ventricle. Ependymomas and choroid plexus papillomas are found at the same location. Surgery and adjunctive therapy are often palliative.[1,10,11]

TABLE 8-1 **Rare Lesions of the Cerebellopontine Angle**

1. Congenital Rest-associated Lesions
   - Cholesteatoma, dermoid, epidermoid
   - Lipoma
   - Respiratory endothelial cyst
   - Enterogenous cyst
   - Choroidal epithelial cyst
   - Salivary gland heterotopia
   - Heteroglial tissue

2. Primary Brainstem Lesions
   - Glioma
   - Astrocytoma
   - Oligodendroglioma
   - Ependymoma
   - Choroid plexus papilloma
   - Glioblastoma multiforme

3. Primary Cerebellar Lesions
   - Medulloblastoma
   - Rhabdomyosarcoma
   - Hemangioblastoma
   - Hemangiosarcoma
   - Glioblastoma multiforme
   - Anaplastic astrocytoma

4. Inflammatory Lesions
   - Arachnoid cyst
   - Cholesterol granuloma of petrous apex
   - Granuloma
   - Focal arachnoiditis

5. Other Cranial Nerve Lesions
   - Trigeminal neuroma
   - Facial nerve neuroma
   - Glossopharyngeal neuroma
   - Vagal neuroma
   - Hypoglossal nerve neuroma

6. Lesions of Direct Extension from Skull Base
   - Glomus tumors
   - Craniopharyngioma
   - Petrous apex cholesteatoma
   - Chondroma
   - Chondrosarcoma
   - Osteosarcoma
   - Adenoma
     - Ceruminous
     - Adenocarcinoma of endolymphatic sac

7. Vascular Lesions
   - Fusiform aneurysm
   - Saccular aneurysm
   - Hemangioma
   - Hemangioblastoma
   - Hemangiosarcoma
   - Hematoma

8. Lesions Metastatic from other Intracranial Neoplasms
   - Craniopharyngioma
   - Pineal gland tumor

9. Metastatic Lesions from Nonintracranial Sources
   - Lung
   - Breast
   - Cervix clear cell adenocarcinoma
   - Pharynx squamous cell carcinoma

10. Malignant Degeneration of Intracranial Congenital Rests
    - Squamous cell carcinoma
    - Melanoma
    - Adenoid cystic carcinoma
    - Malignant teratoma

11. Miscellaneous

Source: Jackler RK, Brackmann DE. Neurotology, 2nd edition. Elsevier/Mosby, Philadelphia, Pennsylvania 19106, 2005. p. 851.

Schwannomas of cranial nerves other the VIII represent 2%–3% of CPA lesions. The most troubling are facial nerve schwannomas, which more often involve the middle cranial fossa. These tumors are slow growing and present with facial nerve paresis and synkinesis. They are rarely malignant and part of neurofibromatosis 2. Diagnosis is based on MRI findings and nerve excitability tests. Because facial nerve function cannot usually be preserved with tumor resection treatment is frequently radiosurgery. Only after the tumor growth results in complete facial paralysis is surgical excision performed. Nerve rerouting with end-to-end anastomosis or cable grafting is performed and supported by fenestrated collagen tubes. The best postoperative outcome is level 3 facial function on the House/Brackmann scale. Trigeminal schwannomas presenting with decreased facial sensation and weak muscles of mastication, and lower cranial nerve schwannomas with wide jugular foramen are managed in similar fashion as acoustic neuromas.[1,6,7,12]

Skull-based neoplasm, such as glomus jugulare, fibrous histiocytomas, and chondromas, may extend to the CPA and require embolization, surgery, or radiation. Papillary endolymphatic lesions associated with von Hippel-Lindau disease and CPA extension usually require surgery.

Vascular lesions (aneurysms and hemangiomas) are diagnosed by MRI, magnetic resonance angiography, magnetic resonance venography, CT, and angiograms. Depending on symptomatology and extent of pathology embolization and surgical excision or clip insertion may be required. Metastatic lesions to the CPA are usually adenocarcinomas of breast or prostate. Lung cancer and melanomas have also been reported with distal metastasis to the CPA and IAC.[1,7,13]

KEY POINTS TO REMEMBER

- Facial nerve preservation is more important than hearing conservation in the treatment plan.
- If there is a facial nerve deficit eye protection is mandatory.
- Unusual lesions of the CPA include lipomas, arachnoid cysts, schwannomas of other cranial nerves, glomus tumors, metastatic lesions, and vascular anomalies.

Further Reading
1. Jackler RK, Brackmann DE. Neurotology, 2nd edition. Elsevier/Mosby, Philadelphia, Pennsylvania 19106, 2005. pp. 850–74.
2. Harnsberger HR, Wiggins III RH, Swartz JD, et al. Epidermoid. In: Temporal Bone-Top 100 Diagnoses. Amirys/W.B. Saunders, Philadelphia, Pennsylvania/Salt Lake City, Utah, 2003. p. 199.
3. Bonneville F, Savatovsky J, Chiras J. Imaging of cerebellopontine angle lesions: an update. Part 2: intra-axial lesions, skull base lesions that may invade the CPA region, and non-enhancing extra-axial lesions. Fur Radiol 2007;17(11):2908–20.
4. Bonnerville F, Sarrazin JL, Mursot-Dupuch K, et al. Unusual lesions of the cerebellopontine angle: a segmental approach. Radiographics 2001;21(2):419–38.
5. Sirin S, Gonul E, Kahraman S, et al. Imaging of posterior fossa epidermoid tumors. Clin Neurol Neurosurg 2005;107(6):461–7.
6. Samii M, Gerganov VM. Tumors of the cerebellopontine angle. Handbook Clin Neurol 2012;105:633–9.
7. Kohan D, Downey L, Lim J, et al. Uncommon lesions presenting as tumors of the internal auditory canal and cerebellopontine angle. Am J Otol 1997;18(3):386–92.
8. Brodsky JR, Smith TW, Litofsky S, et al. Lipoma of the cerebellopontine angle. Am J Otolaryngol 2006;27(4):271–4.
9. Gonul E, Izci Y, Onguru O. Arachnoid cyst of the cerebellopontine angle associated with gliosis of the eighth cranial nerve. J Clin Neurosci 2007;14(7):700–2.
10. Wu B, Liu W, Zhu H, et al. Primary glioblastoma of the cerebellopontine angle in adults. J Neurosur 2011;114(5):1288–93.
11. Spina A, Boari N, Gaghardi F, et al. Review of cerebellopontine angle medulloblastoma. Br J Neurosurg 2012. PMID:23163297.
12. Sherman JD, Dagnew E, Pensak ML, et al. Facial nerve neuromas: report of 10 cases and review of the literature. Neurosurgery 2002;50(3):450–6.
13. Hariharan S, Zhu J, Nadkarni MA, et al. Metastatic lung cancer in the cerebellopontine angles mimicking bilateral acoustic neuroma. J Clin Neurosci 2005;12(2):184–6.

SECTION II
Vertigo and Dysequilibrium

9 Ménière's Disease

A 42-year-old female presents for evaluation of vertigo. She states that this has been a problem episodically for the past 6 months. She has had seven episodes over this time period. She describes the sensation of true horizontal axis vertigo lasting anywhere from 30 minutes to 3 hours. There is associated severe nausea and emesis. She denies any preceding history of headache, photophobia, or phonophobia. Immediately prior to each vertigo episode she experiences the sensation of pressure and fullness in her left ear. There is associated roaring tinnitus in the left ear immediately prior to and during the episodes of vertigo and a mild hearing loss. Past medical history is significant for seasonal allergies. There is no past surgical or trauma history. Medications include oral contraceptive and an antihistamine. As for social history, she does not use tobacco. She consumes one to two glasses of red wine weekly. She denies recreational drug use. She consumes six to seven cups of caffeinated beverages daily including coffee and soda. Her daily sodium consumption is greater than 4,000 mg/day, and she consumes less than one glass of water per day. Physical examination is unremarkable. Her most recent audiometric examination is presented in Figure 9-1. Videonystagmography revealed a 30% weakness on the left side. Electrocochleography reveal an abnormally high left summating potential to action potential ratio of 0.6.

What do you do now?

Ménière's disease, also known as idiopathic endolymphatic hydrops, is a relatively common cause of vertigo. It is the etiologic factor in approximately 10% of patients presenting for evaluation of vertigo.[1,2] The incidence of Ménière's disease is estimated to range from approximately 15 to 45 per 100,000 in most studies with a prevalence of approximately 220 per 100,000.[2-5] Ménière's disease is a disease process involving the inner ear with an associated finding of fluid imbalance in the inner ear (hydrops). The clinical significance of hydrops in Ménière's disease has become controversial. Traditionally, hydrops was believed to be the pathophysiologic factor precipitating the symptoms observed in Ménière's disease. However, recent studies have revealed that hydrops alone is not sufficient to produce the characteristic symptoms associated with Ménière's disease.[6] The exact etiology of Ménière's disease is not understood. Hydrops is a feature of the disease presentation, but may not entirely be the causative factor. It is currently postulated that the etiology of Ménière's disease is multifactorial with observed allergic, immunologic, autoimmune, and viral etiologic associations.[7,8]

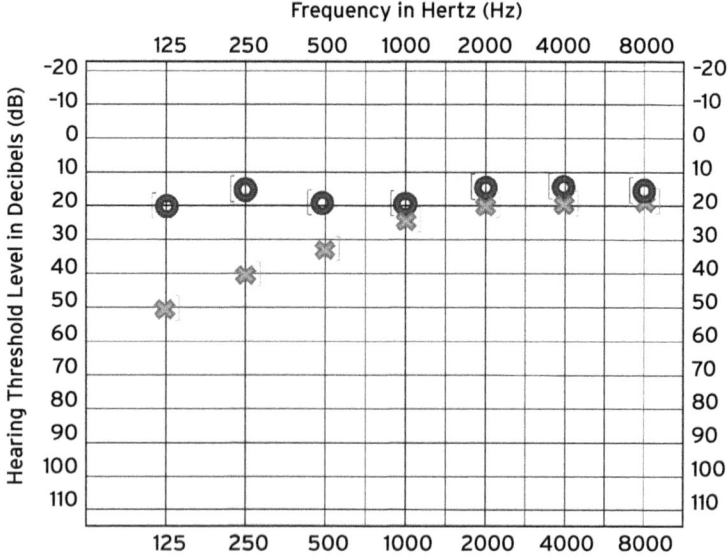

FIGURE 9-1 Pure tone audiogram from patient with episodic vertigo, tinnitus, aural fullness, and hearing loss.

Ménière's disease typically presents as unilateral disease; however, in approximately 10% of patients bilateral presentation may be observed.[9-11] Additionally, greater than 40% of patients throughout the course of disease progress to bilateral involvement.[9-11]

Although Ménière's disease may present at almost any age, the peak prevalence is between ages 40 and 60 years.[2,12] A slight female preponderance for disease has been observed.[2,9] Additionally a familial association has been reported in 10%–20% of affected individuals.[13]

Ménière's disease is characterized by a classic tetrad of symptoms; however, variants of disease have been described within the literature. The classic tetrad of symptoms associated with Ménière's disease includes:

- Intermittent episodic vertigo (true horizontal axis spinning sensation)
- Fluctuating hearing loss
- Tinnitus (low-tone roaring)
- Aural fullness (pressure or fullness sensation in the affected ear)

Variants including cochlear Ménière's disease (characterized by fluctuating hearing loss alone) or vestibular Ménière's disease (characterized by episodic vertigo alone) have been described. These patients, however, typically progress to classic Ménière's disease throughout their clinical course.[14,15] To clarify the diagnosis and unify the reporting of Ménière's disease, the Committee on Hearing and Equilibrium of the American Academy of Otolaryngology–Head and Neck Surgery authored diagnostic criteria for Ménière's disease (Table 9-1).[16]

CLINICAL PRESENTATION

The diagnosis of Ménière's disease is largely based on patient history. Thus, a clear and detailed description of the episodes in question is of critical importance in evaluating these patients. Patients presenting with Ménière's disease present with true horizontal axis vertigo or subjective sensation of motion. On clinical evaluation, these patients are noted to have horizontal or rotatory nystagmus during acute episodes of vertigo.[16] The vertigo episodes typically last for minutes to hours with associated nausea and emesis. Patients may additionally present with diaphoresis or pallor. The episodes of vertigo are classically preceded by Lermoyez attacks (increased tinnitus

TABLE 9-1 **Committee on Hearing and Equilibrium of the American Academy of Otolaryngology–Head and Neck Surgery Diagnostic Criteria for Ménière's Disease**

Diagnosis of Ménière's Disease

Certain Ménière's disease

Definite Ménière's disease, plus histopathologic confirmation

Definite Ménière's disease

Two or more definitive spontaneous episodes of vertigo lasting 20 minutes or longer

Audiometrically documented hearing loss on at least one occasion

Tinnitus or aural fullness in the treated ear

Other causes excluded

Probable Ménière's disease

One definitive episode of vertigo

Audiometrically documented hearing loss on at least one occasion

Tinnitus or aural fullness in the treated ear

Other causes excluded

Possible Ménière's disease

Episodic vertigo of the Ménière's type without documented hearing loss, or

Sensorineural hearing loss, fluctuating or fixed, with dysequilibrium but without definite episodes

Other causes excluded

Source: Monsell EM. New and revised reporting guidelines for the Committee on Hearing and Equilibrium. American Academy of Otolaryngology–Head and Neck Surgery Foundation, Inc. *Otolaryngol Head Neck Surg* 1995;113:176–8.

and sensorineural hearing loss preceding onset of vertigo).[17] The episodes of vertigo vary in intensity by episode and by patient. Certain triggers have been identified that may precipitate attacks of vertigo including menses, psychosocial stress, and certain dietary consumptions.

Hearing loss is typically associated with acute attacks of vertigo. During acute episodes, low-frequency hearing loss may be experienced. At initial presentation, episodes of hearing loss tend to be fluctuating. However, as the disease process progresses, hearing loss may become permanent and progressive. Similarly, tinnitus typically occurs with episodes of vertigo and may too become constant. The severity of hearing loss and tinnitus, like vertigo, is highly variable among individuals suffering from Ménière's disease.

In a distinct subset of patients, drop attacks may be experienced. These attacks, known as Tumarkin attacks or crises of Tumarkin, are episodes in which patients experience sudden falls without loss of consciousness.[18] Tumarkin attacks present in less than 10% of patients with Ménière's disease and tend to present as clustered events.

During acute vertigo attacks, patients tend to present in distress with associated nystagmus, diaphoresis, pallor, nausea, and emesis often initially precipitating a visit to the emergency department. However, the challenge in diagnosing Ménière's disease is that in the initial course of disease between acute episodes, patients tend to present asymptomatically with no significant clinical findings. It is therefore important to again stress the importance of keen assessment of the clinical history when evaluating patients with attacks of vertigo in the outpatient setting.

DIAGNOSTIC EVALUATION

The diagnostic evaluation of patients with episodic vertigo with a suspicion for Ménière's disease should include an audiometric evaluation. Pure tone audiometry, speech discrimination score, tympanometry, and acoustic reflexes should be performed. During the early phase of disease between episodes normal hearing may be observed. The finding of normal hearing does not preclude the diagnosis of Ménière's disease. During acute episodes in the early phase of disease, patients may present with a threshold shift, typically in the low frequencies, and a decline in speech discrimination scores. Acoustic reflexes and tympanometry should be normal in all phases of disease. This threshold shift in the early phase tends to be transient with return to normal hearing between episodes. Over time decline in hearing may become progressive and permanent.

Traditionally, glycerol or furosemide test was performed during acute attacks. During glycerol or furosemide testing, audiometric evaluation is performed during an acute attack of Ménière's disease to evaluate for acute auditory threshold shifts. The patients are then administered either of these agents during the acute attacks. Improvement in word recognition score of 16% or improvement in pure tone threshold by 25 dB at three frequencies following administration of agent is deemed positive test for Ménière's disease. These tests, however, have lost favor in that they are difficult to coordinate and poorly tolerated by patients. Thus, they are rarely performed.

Electrophysiologic studies including electronystagmography or videonystagmography may be performed to assess the relative functionality of the vestibular labyrinth, namely the horizontal semicircular canal. Temperature changes in the horizontal semicircular canal are induced by cold and warm air or water instilled into the external auditory canal inducing a characteristic nystagmus response. Asymmetry in function can be detected by differences in nystagmus recorded either by electrical or video assessment. Hyperfunction or hypofunction may be observed in the affected ear depending on the phase of disease. Approximately 50%–75% of patients with Ménière's disease exhibit an asymmetry on this testing with 6%–11% of patients exhibiting a complete loss of function.[19]

The most sensitive test for Ménière's disease currently available is electrocochleography. This test is an electrophysiologic study that measures summating potential (related to movement of the basilar membrane) and the nerve action potential. A ratio greater than 0.4 is indicative of a hydroptic state.

In a patient with symptoms lacking the characteristic presentation of Ménière's disease, imaging of the cerebellopontine angle including magnetic resonance imaging or electrophysiologic studies including auditory brainstem response testing may be performed to evaluate for pathology involving the internal auditory canal or cerebellopontine angle. Table 9-2 presents a differential diagnosis for patient presenting with episodic vertigo. These entities within the differential diagnosis should be ruled out either by history, physical examination findings, or further studies before the diagnosis of Ménière's disease is made.

NATURAL HISTORY

The natural history of Ménière's disease is one of spontaneous remission in most patients. At 2 years, more than 50% of patients experience spontaneous remission of disease. By 8 years, this number increases to greater than

TABLE 9-2 **Differential Diagnosis for Ménière's Disease**

Differential Diagnosis

Autoimmune disease	Salicylate toxicity
Barre-Lieou syndrome	Temporal bone malignancy
Basilar artery thrombosis	Temporal lobe epilepsy
Basilar meningitis	Thyroid dysfunction
Cogan syndrome	Toxic vestibular injury
Congenital anomalies	Transient ischemic attack
Diabetes	Trauma
Electrolyte imbalance	Tumor of cerebellopontine angle
Endocrine abnormalities	Vascular infarct
Hyperlipidemia	Vasculitis
Labyrinthitis	Vestibular neuronitis
Otosclerosis	Viral meningitis
Perilymphatic fistula	Wernicke encephalopathy

70%.[2,20] However, despite spontaneous remission, patients often experience permanent vestibular deficits and hearing decline.

TREATMENT

During acute episodes vestibular suppressants (i.e., meclizine, diazepam) may be of assistance in abating acute attacks of vertigo, but these agents are not recommended for long-term preventive therapy in Ménière's disease. Because of the high rate of spontaneous remission, conservative therapies should be explored and exhausted to manage and prevent attacks. Dietary restriction including low sodium intake (less than 1.5 g/day), restriction of chocolate, and caffeine avoidance should be used. In patients failing conservative dietary restriction, diuretics have been demonstrated to be of great benefit in most patients.[21,22]

The Meniette device has been advocated by certain clinicians in the management of Ménière's disease. The Meniette device requires placement of a pressure equalization tube allowing for pressure pulses to be delivered to the inner ear. The mechanism of action of the Meniette device is not well understood; however, it has been found to provide symptomatic relief with daily use in limited studies.[23,24]

Approximately 5%–10% of patients with Ménière's disease ultimately require operative management for control of disease. Surgical management of Ménière's disease includes both nonablative and ablative procedures. The goal of a nonablative procedure is to decrease or alleviate attacks of vertigo while maintaining the residual functionality of the vestibular labyrinth. Nonablative procedures include endolymphatic sac decompression or intratympanic steroid instillation. Endolymphatic sac decompression has been demonstrated to exhibit immediate success in up to 75% of patients.[25] Intratympanic steroid instillation is gaining favor in the treatment of acute episodes of vertigo and preventing progression of disease.[26] In cases where nonablative therapies have been unsuccessful ablative therapies that do not preserve the functional integrity of the vestibular labyrinth may be used. These therapies include chemical ablation (i.e., intratympanic gentamicin injection), labyrinthectomy, or vestibular nerve sectioning. Success rates of approximately 90% have been reported with both chemical and surgical ablation.[27]

> **KEY POINTS TO REMEMBER**
>
> - Ménière's disease is believed to be associated with endolymphatic hydrops
> - Sodium restriction and diuretics are first-line therapy
> - Steroids have shown promise in treatment of Ménière's disease
> - Blacking out or loss of consciousness is NOT associated with Ménière's disease and should prompt further investigation

Further Reading
1. Bhattacharyya N, Baugh RF, Orvidas L, et al. Clinical practice guideline: benign paroxysmal positional vertigo. Otolaryngol Head Neck Surg 2008;139:S47–81.
2. Minor LB, Schessel DA, Carey JP. Ménière's disease. Curr Opin Neurol 2004;17:9–16.

3. Stahle J, Stahl C, Arenberg IK. Incidence of Ménière's disease. Arch Otolaryngol 1978;104:99–102.
4. Wilmot TJ. Meniere's disease: a review. Clin Otolaryngol 1979;4:131–43.
5. Wladislavosky-Wasserman P, Facer GW, Mokri B, et al. Meniere's disease: a 30 year epidemiologic and clinical study in Rochester, MA, 1951–80. Laryngoscope 1984;94:1098–102.
6. Merchant SN, Adams JC, Nadol JB Jr. Pathophysiology of Meniere's syndrome: are symptoms caused by endolymphatic hydrops? Otol Neurotol 2005;26:74–81.
7. Greco A, Gallo A, Fusconi M, et al. Meniere's disease might be an autoimmune condition? Autoimmun Rev 2012;11:731–8.
8. Derbery MJ. Allergic and immunologic features of Ménière's disease. Otolaryngol Clin North Am 2011;44:655–66.
9. Balkany T, Sizes B, Arenberg I. Bilateral aspects of Ménière's disease: an underestimated clinical entity. Otolaryngol Clin North Am 1980;13:603–9.
10. Green JD Jr, Blum DJ, Harner SG. Longitudinal follow-up of patients with Meniere's disease. Otolaryngol Head Neck Surg 1991;104:783–8.
11. Kitahara M. Bilateral aspects of Ménière's disease. Ménière's disease with bilateral fluctuant hearing loss. Acta Otolaryngol Suppl 1991;485:74–7.
12. Paparella MM. The cause (multifactorial inheritance) and pathogenesis (endolymphatic malabsorption) of Ménière's disease and its symptoms (mechanical and chemical). Acta Otolaryngol (Stockh) 1985;99:445–51.
13. Morris AW. Anticipation in Ménière's disease. J Laryngol Otol 1995;109:499–502.
14. Kitahara M, Takeda T, Yazawa Y, et al. Pathophysiology of Meniere's disease and it subvarieties. Acta Otolaryngol Suppl 1984;406:52–5.
15. Paparella MM, Mancini F. Vestibular Ménière's disease. Otolaryngol Head Neck Surg 1985;93:148–51.
16. Monsell EM. New and revised reporting guidelines for the Committee on Hearing and Equilibrium. American Academy of Otolaryngology–Head and Neck Surgery Foundation, Inc. Otolaryngol Head Neck Surg 1995;113:176–8.
17. Lermoyez M. Le vertige qui fait entendre (angiospasme labyrinthique). Presse Med 1919:27:1–3.
18. Baloh RW, Jacobson K, Winder T. Drop attacks with Ménière's syndrome. Ann Neurol 1990;28:384–7.
19. Black O, Kitch R. A review of vestibular test results in Meniere's disease. Otolaryngol Clin North Am 1980;13:631–42.
20. Silverstein H, Smouha E, Jones R. Natural history vs. surgery for Meniere's disease. Otolaryngol Head Neck Surg 1989;100:6–16.
21. Klockhoff I, Lindblom U. Meniere's disease and hydrochlorothiazide: a critical analysis of symptoms and therapeutic effects. Acta Otolaryngol (Stockh) 1967;63:347–65.
22. Klockhoff I, Lindblom U, Stahle J. Diuretic treatment of Meniere's disease. Acta Otolaryngol 1974;100:262–5.

23. Barbara M, Consagra C, Monini S, et al. Local pressure protocol, including Meniett, in the treatment of Meniere's disease: short-term results during the active stage. Acta Otolaryngol 2001;121:939–44.
24. Gates GA, Green D. Intermittent pressure therapy of intractable Meniere's disease using the Meniett device: a preliminary report. Laryngoscope 2002;112:1489–93.
25. Arenberg IK. Results of endolymphatic sac to mastoid shunt surgery for Meniere's disease refractory to medical therapy. Am J Otol 1987;8:271.
26. Phillips JS, Westerberg B. Intratympanic steroids for Meniere's disease or syndrome. Cochran Database Syst Rev 2011;7:CD008514.
27. Schmerber S, Dumas G, Morel N, et al. Vestibular neurectomy vs. chemical labyrinthectomy in the treatment of disabling Ménière's disease: a long-term comparative study. Auris Nasus Larynx 2009;36:400–5.

10 Vestibular Neuropathy

A 53-year-old male presents for evaluation of vertigo. His vertigo is continuous and unremitting. The vertigo has been ongoing for the past 5 days. He was initially seen in the emergency department and instructed to follow-up with a specialist if symptoms do not abate. Diazepam prescribed in the emergency department temporarily improves symptoms. He denies any associated hearing loss, tinnitus, aural fullness, headache, photophobia, or phonophobia. He does report nausea and emesis with severe intensity of symptoms. There is no history of head trauma. He had a recent upper respiratory tract infection during the preceding week. His past medical and surgical history is significant for hypertension and hyperlipidemia. His medications include a β-blocker and statin medication. He smoked 10 cigarettes per day for the past 30 years. He consumes three to five mixed alcoholic drinks per week and denies recreational drug use. He drinks one to two cups of caffeinated beverages daily and two to four glasses of water. The physical examination is significant for an obese male who appears his stated age. He is noted to have horizontal nystagmus with the fast-phase beating toward the right. Head shake test reveals augmented nystagmus. Cranial nerve and neurologic examination including Romberg is otherwise normal. The patient had a normal otologic examination including tuning fork tests. The remainder of the examination was within normal limits. Audiometric evaluation was normal (Figure 10-1). His speech discrimination scores were 100% bilaterally. Tympanograms were type A bilaterally, and the patient was noted to have normal acoustic reflexes.

What do you do now?

The term vestibular neuronitis was first coined by Dix and Hallpike in 1952.[1,2] Since that time, this pathology has also become known as idiopathic acute vestibular dysfunction, vestibular neuritis, and less commonly vestibular ganglionitis. Vestibular neuronitis is the second most common cause of vertigo. The annual incidence of vestibular neuronitis is approximately 3.5 per 100,000 population.[3,4] Vestibular neuronitis is estimated to account for 3%–10% of patients seeking medical attention in specialty clinic for vertigo.[5,6] The etiology of vestibular neuronitis is not well understood. Microvascular disease resulting in ischemia of the vestibular nerve has been postulated.[7] Alternatively, an infectious etiology has long been proposed.[1,2] An association with viral upper respiratory tract infections has been identified.[8,9] Viral agents have been proposed as the etiologic factor involved in the vestibular neuronitis; multiple studies have identified latent herpes simplex virus 1 as an associated factor in vestibular neuronitis.[10-15] Vestibular neuronitis may occur at any age but has a peak prevalence among individuals between the ages of 30 and 50 years.[1,2,4] There is no gender predilection associated with this disease process.

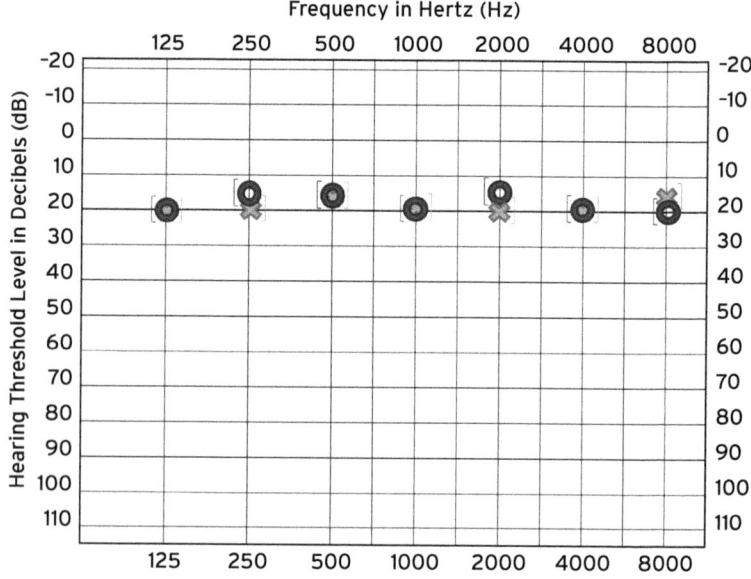

FIGURE 10-1 Pure audiogram from patient with 5 days of continuous vertigo.

CLINICAL PRESENTATION

The diagnosis of vestibular neuronitis is largely based on the history and clinical presentation. Patients presenting with vestibular neuronitis typically present with the following symptoms:

- Vertigo (true horizontal axis rotatory)
- Nausea and emesis
- Normal or unchanged hearing
- No additional neurologic findings

The onset of vertigo is sudden in most patients; however, in a small minority of patients, onset may be progressive with preceding dizziness or dysequilibrium. During the acute phase, symptoms of vertigo may be quite severe. Vertigo may last for several hours to days during an episode of vestibular neuronitis. Patients may report that symptoms of vertigo are exacerbated by movement. Hearing loss is not associated with vestibular neuronitis; thus, the complaint of hearing loss in association with severe sudden onset of vertigo directs the clinical suspicion away from a diagnosis of vestibular neuronitis. Similarly, loss of consciousness, weakness, paresthesias, paresis, or headache are not associated with vestibular neuronitis. The presence of these symptoms should prompt further investigation into the etiology of these symptoms.

During the latent phase of vestibular neuronitis, symptoms of vertigo abate. However, patients may report dysequilibrium, imbalance, or unsteadiness, which may remain for several weeks following the episode of vestibular neuronitis. Interestingly, patients often also report feeling heady in their head or simply feeling "off" for days to weeks after the initial episode.[6]

DIAGNOSTIC EVALUATION

As stated previously, the diagnosis of vestibular neuronitis is based largely on clinical presentation. However, there are certain findings on physical examination that support the diagnosis. A complete head and neck and neurologic examination should be performed in the evaluation of patients with a clinical suspicion of vestibular neuronitis. During the acute phase of disease, patients with vestibular neuronitis typically present with horizontal or rotatory nystagmus, which may be either spontaneous or gaze induced. Head thrust examination and head shake examination may induce nystagmus or augment spontaneous nystagmus.[16] Tuning fork examination should also be performed to assess for asymmetry in hearing. In patients with vestibular neuronitis, the Weber examination is midline unless the patient has preexisting asymmetries in hearing. The Rinne examination is positive (i.e., air conduction greater than bone conduction). The remainder of the physical examination typically is within normal limits. The presence of additional neurologic findings on examination should prompt further evaluation and clinical suspicion of an alternative diagnosis.

The diagnostic evaluation of vestibular neuronitis is typically conservative. Audiometric evaluation including pure tone audiometry, speech discrimination testing, tympanometry, and acoustic reflexes is not typically performed in the diagnosis of vestibular neuronitis. However, audiometric evaluation may be of benefit in confirming normal hearing or lack of acute changes in hearing in patients with preexisting audiometric abnormalities. Similarly, vestibular testing, including electronystagmography, videonystagmography, or vestibular evoked myogenic potentials, is typically not performed in the diagnostic evaluation of vestibular neuronitis. However, if the diagnosis of vestibular neuronitis is uncertain, further vestibular testing may be of benefit. Additionally, imaging is not typically required. However, if there is uncertainty regarding the diagnosis, temporal bone or posterior fossa imaging should be obtained.

The differential diagnosis of vestibular neuronitis is quite extensive. The following disease processes should be considered within the differential of patients presenting with acute onset of vertigo:

- Brainstem hemorrhage
- Brainstem ischemia
- Cerebellar hemorrhage
- Cerebellar ischemia
- Labyrinthitis
- Ménière's disease
- Multiple sclerosis
- Ototoxin exposure
- Perilymphatic fistula/traumatic disruption of the otic capsule

		Hearing Loss	
		Yes	No
Episodic	Yes	Ménière's Disease	BPPV
	No	Labyrinthitis	Vestibular Neuronitis

FIGURE 10-2 Four most common causes of peripheral vertigo. BPPV, benign paroxysmal positional vertigo.

- Tumors of the internal auditory canal, brainstem, or cerebellopontine angle
- Vertebral artery dissection
- Vertebrobasilar insufficiency

Additionally, Figure 10-2 presents the four most common causes of peripheral vertigo. The hallmark of vestibular neuronitis as compared with most other disease processes included within the differential is the lack of hearing loss or additional neurologic findings. A thorough and detailed history and physical examination is of critical importance in diagnosing vestibular neuronitis.

NATURAL HISTORY

Vestibular neuronitis is a self-limiting disease process. Symptoms of vertigo typically resolve within hours to days on onset with residual dysequilibrium and instability resolving within weeks following the episode. Recurrence has been reported in approximately 2% of patients in most series.[17,18] However, higher rates of recurrence have been reported.[19] Interestingly, vestibular neuronitis has been associated with an increased risk of developing benign paroxysmal positional vertigo. This occurs in approximately 10%–15% of patients following vestibular neuronitis.[17-19] The pathophysiology of this association is not well understood, but has been postulated to be secondary to loosening of the utricular otoconia with the episode of neuronitis[20] or vascular injury.[21] Following vestibular neuronitis, posterior canal benign paroxysmal positional vertigo, also known as Lindsay-Hemenway syndrome, is more commonly reported.[18]

TREATMENT

Because the natural history of vestibular neuronitis is one of self-limited disease, the care of patients with vestibular neuronitis is largely supportive. Antiemetics may be prescribed to reduce associated nausea and emesis. In extreme cases, intravenous hydration may be required for hyperemesis. Within the acute phase, vestibular suppressants are of benefit in reducing severe vertigo until its spontaneous resolution. The use of vestibular suppressants should be limited to a short course and should not be used for treatment of latent symptoms of dysequilibrium because it may compromise central vestibular compensation. Antiviral therapy has no effect on outcomes in patients with vestibular neuronitis.[22] Similarly, despite early reports of effect,[22] corticosteroids have not revealed a significant clinical impact on outcomes in these patients.[23,24]

Most patients following an episodes of vestibular neuronitis retain some degree of permanent vestibular hypofunction.[16,25] Vestibular therapy performed by dedicated vestibular therapists has been demonstrated to be of benefit in facilitating compensation of unilateral vestibular hypofunction following an episode of vestibular neuronitis.[6,26-29] Surgical management including vestibular nerve sectioning is reserved for patients with severe chronic symptoms not improved by an extended course of vestibular rehabilitation and has been demonstrated to be of great benefit.[6,30,31]

> **KEY POINTS TO REMEMBER**
>
> - Vestibular neuropathy does not have associated hearing loss
> - Treatment is supportive
> - Disease is typically self-limited

Further Reading

1. Dix M, Hallpike C. The pathology, symptomatology, and diagnosis of certain common disorders of the vestibular system. Ann Otol Rhinol Laryngol 1952;61:987–1016.
2. Dix M, Hallpike C. The pathology, symptomatology, and diagnosis of certain common disorders of the vestibular system. Proc R Soc Med 1952;45:341–54.
3. Strupp M, Brandt T. Vestibular neuritis. Semi Neurol 2009;29:509–19.
4. Sekitani T, Imate Y, Noguchi T, et al. Vestibular neuronitis: epidemiological survey by questionnaire in Japan. Acta Otolaryngol Suppl 1993;503:9–12.
5. Neuhauser H. Epidemiology of vertigo. Curr Opin Neurol 2007;20:40–6.
6. Goddard JC, Fayad JN. Vestibular neuritis. Otolaryngol Clin N Am 2011;44:361–5.
7. Nadol JB Jr. Vestibular neuritis. Otolaryngol Head Neck Surg 1995;112:162–72.
8. Coats AC. Vestibular neuronitis. Trans Am Acad Ophthalmol Otolaryngol 1969;73:395–408.
9. Davis LE. Viruses and vestibular neuritis: review of human and animal studies. Acta Otolaryngol Suppl 1993;503:70–3.
10. Schuknecht HF, Kitamura K. Second Louis H Clerf Lecture. Vestibular neuritis. Ann Otol Rhinol Laryngol Suppl 1981;90:1–19.
11. Furata Y, Takasu T, Fukuda S, et al. Latent herpes simplex virus 1 in human vestibular ganglia. Acta Otolaryngol Suppl 1993;503:85–9.
12. Hirata Y, Gyo K, Yanagihara N. Herpetic vestibular neuritis: an experimental study. Acta Otolaryngol Suppl 1995;519:93–6.
13. Gacek R, Gacek M. The three faces of vestibular ganglionitis. Ann Otol Rhinol Laryngol 2002;111:103–14.
14. Theil D, Arbusow V, Deurfuss T, et al. Prevalence of HSV-1 LAT in human trigeminal, geniculate, and vestibular ganglia and its implication for cranial nerve syndromes. Brain Pathol 2001;11:408–13.
15. Baloh RW, Ishiyama A, Wackym P, et al. Vestibular neuritis: clinical-pathological correlation. Otolaryngol Head Neck Surg 1996;114:586–92.
16. Choi KD, Oh SY, Kim HJ, et al. Recovery of vestibular imbalances after vestibular neuritis. Laryngoscope 2007;117:1307–12.
17. Huppert D, Strupp M, Theil D, et al. Low recurrence rate of vestibular neuritis: a long-term follow-up. Neurology 2006;67:1870–1.
18. Mandala M, Santoro GP, Awrey J, Nuti D. Vestibular neuritis: recurrence and incidence of secondary benign paroxysmal positional vertigo. Acta Otolarngol 2010;130:565–7.
19. Kim YH, Kim KS, Kim KJ, et al. Recurrence of vertigo in patient with vestibular neuritis. Acta Otolaryngol 2011;131:1172–7.
20. Schuknecht HF. Positional vertigo: clinical and experimental observations. Trans Am Acad Opthalmol Otolaryngol 1962;66:319–31.
21. Pardal Refoyo JL, Perez Plasencia D, Beltran Mateos LD. Ischemia of the anterior vestibular artery (Lindsay-Hemenway syndrome). Acta Otorrinolaringol Esp 1998;49:599–602.

22. Strupp M, Zingler VC, Arbusow V, et al. Methylprednisolone, valacyclovir, or the combination for vestibular neuritis. N Engl J Med 2004;351:354–61.
23. Fishman JM, Burgess C, Waddell A. Corticosteroids for the treatment of idiopathic acute vestibular dysfunction (vestibular neuritis). Cochrane Database Syst Rev 2011;5:CD008607.
24. Fishman JM. Corticosteroids effective in idiopathic facial nerve palsy (Bell's palsy) but not necessarily in idiopathic acute vestibular dysfunction (vestibular neuritis). Laryngoscope 2011;121:2494–5.
25. Baloh RW. Clinical practice. Vestibular neuritis. N Engl J Med 2003;348:1027–32.
26. Alrwaily W, Whitney SL. Vestibular rehabilitation of older adults with dizziness. Otolaryngol Clin North Am 2011;44:473–96.
27. Strupp M, Arbusow V, Maag KP, et al. Vestibular exercises improve central vestibulospinal compensation after vestibular neuritis. Neurology 1998;51:838–44.
28. Komazec Z, Lemajic S. [Specific vestibular exercises in the treatment of vestibular neuritis]. Med Pregl 2004;57:269–74.
29. Whitney SL, Rossi MM. Efficacy of vestibular rehabilitation. Otolaryngol Clin North Am 2000;33:659–72.
30. Benecke JE. Surgery for non-Meniere's vertigo. Acta Otolaryngol Suppl 1994;513:37–9.
31. Pappas D, Pappas D. Vestibular nerve section: long-term follow-up. Laryngoscope 1997;107:1203–9.

11 Labyrinthitis

A 48-year-old female presents for evaluation of vertigo and hearing loss. Her vertigo is continuous and unremitting for the past 5 days. She reports significant loss of hearing on the right, but states that she is still able to hear a dial tone on the telephone. She is unable to understand the speech of individuals talking on the telephone in her right ear. She was initially seen in the emergency department; given meclizine and diazepam, which temporarily helped; and instructed to follow-up with a specialist within a week. She denies aural fullness but has mild taste disturbance. She denies facial weakness or spasms, headache, photophobia, or phonophobia. She does report intermittent severe nausea and emesis. There is no history of head trauma. She had an upper respiratory tract infection during the preceding week. Her past medical history is significant for type 2 diabetes mellitus and obesity. Her medications include glyburide and a multivitamin. She denies tobacco, ethanol, and recreational drug use. She consumes one to two cups of caffeinated beverages daily. The physical examination is significant for an obese female who appears her stated age. She is noted to have horizontal nystagmus with the fast-phase beating toward the right. Head shake test reveals augmented nystagmus. The neurologic examination including Romberg is otherwise normal. The patient had a normal otologic examination with the exception of the tuning fork examination. The Weber lateralizes to the left. Rinne is positive (air conduction greater than bone conduction) bilaterally. The remainder of the examination was within normal limits. Audiometric evaluation revealed a moderate sloping to severe asymmetric right sensorineural hearing loss (Figure 11-1). Her speech discrimination score was 100% on the left and 68% on the right. Tympanograms were type A bilaterally, and the patient was noted to have normal acoustic reflexes on the right with mild elevation on the left.

What do you do now?

Labyrinthitis is a disease process characterized by inflammation of the inner ear. The etiology of labyrinthitis is most commonly viral or bacterial; however, autoimmune labyrinthitis (i.e., Wegener's granulomatosis or polyarteritis nodosa associated labyrinthitis) has been described. Pathogens associated with the etiology of labyrinthitis are listed in Table 11-1. Viral labyrinthitis is currently the most common form of labyrinthitis. Viral labyrinthitis has most commonly been associated with cytomegalovirus or measles infections. Because of the anatomic associations, bacterial forms of labyrinthitis may be a complication of meningitis or otitis media. As such, bacterial pathogens associated with bacterial labyrinthitis are the same as those commonly associated with otitis media and meningitis. Bacteria-associated labyrinthitis may take the form of suppurative labyrinthitis or serous labyrinthitis. Suppurative labyrinthitis, although rare because of widespread use of antibiotics, may develop by bacterial spread through cerebrospinal fluid to the labyrinth via the internal auditory canal or cochlear aqueduct or from meningitis or in association with otomastoiditis by direct bacterial spread through a dehiscence in the horizontal semicircular canal.[1] Alternatively, serous labyrinthitis occurs more

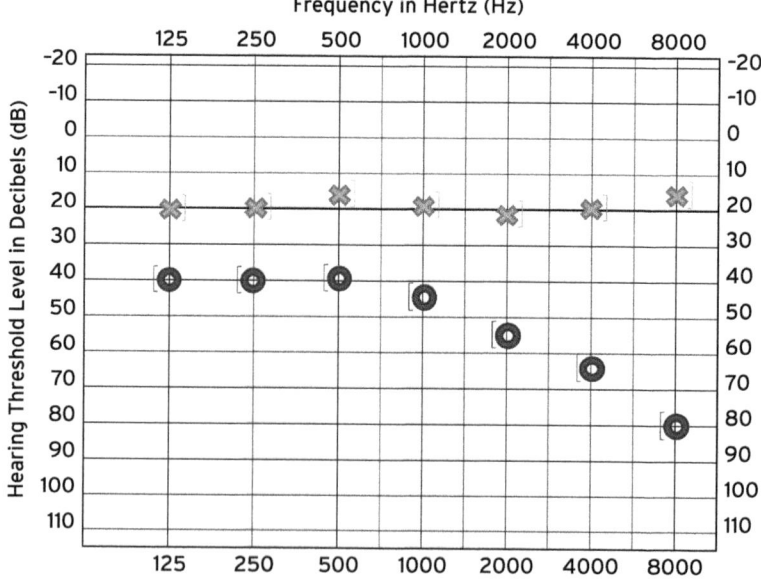

FIGURE 11-1 Pure tone audiogram from patient with unremitting vertigo and hearing loss.

TABLE 11-1 **Pathogens Causing Labyrinthitis**

Pathogens in Labyrinthitis	
Viral Pathogens	Bacterial Pathogens
■ Adenovirus	■ *Bacteroides* species
■ Coxsackievirus	■ *Escherichia coli*
■ Cytomegalovirus	■ *Haemophilus influenzae*
■ Herpes simplex virus 1	■ *Moraxella catarrhalis*
■ Influenza virus	■ *Mycobacterium tuberculosis*
■ Mumps virus	■ *Neisseria meningitidis*
■ Parainfluenza virus	■ *Proteus* species
■ Respiratory syncytial virus	■ *Staphylococcus* species
■ Rubella virus	■ *Streptococcus pneumoniae*
■ Rubeola virus	■ *Streptococcus* species
■ Varicella-zoster virus	

commonly in association with otitis media as a response to bacterial toxins and host inflammatory mediators entering the labyrinth via the round window causing inflammation of the labyrinth.[2] Various changes within the labyrinth have been identified histopathologically in association with labyrinthitis including cochleosaccular degeneration, endolymphatic hydrops, atrophy, fibrosis, or fibro-osseous proliferation in the sensoriepithelia and support cells with secondary neuronal degeneration.[3,4] This translates to various clinical symptoms expressed by patients on presentation and evaluation.

CLINICAL PRESENTATION

The diagnosis of labyrinthitis is largely based on the history and clinical presentation and is quite similar to that of vestibular neuronitis. The distinguishing feature of labyrinthitis on clinical presentation is the presence of associated hearing loss. Patients with labyrinthitis may present with a variety of symptoms including

- Vertigo (true horizontal axis rotatory)
- Nausea and emesis
- Hearing loss
- Tinnitus
- Aural fullness
- Otorrhea
- Otalgia
- Fever
- Facial paresis

The associated symptomatology is largely dependent on the etiologic factor. However, the hallmark symptoms of labyrinthitis are sudden onset, nonepisodic vertigo, and hearing loss. Patients with labyrinthitis present with associated complaints of hearing loss that may range from mild to profound sensorineural hearing loss. Vertigo in association with labyrinthitis is typically of sudden onset. Similar to vestibular neuronitis, during the acute phase, symptoms of vertigo may be quite severe lasting several hours to days. Motion may exacerbate symptoms of vertigo in these patients. On resolution of continuous vertigo, patients often complaint of prolonged dizziness, dysequilibrium, or unsteadiness that may last for weeks to months following onset of disease. However, complaints of loss of consciousness, weakness, paresthesias, paresis, or headache are not associated with labyrinthitis and should direct the clinical suspicion toward an alternative diagnosis. The presence of these symptoms should prompt further investigation into the etiology of these symptoms.

DIAGNOSTIC EVALUATION

Similar to the diagnosis of vestibular neuronitis, the diagnosis of labyrinthitis is largely dependent on clinical presentation. Nevertheless, a complete head and neck and neurologic examination should be performed, which may reveal findings of horizontal or rotatory nystagmus that may be either spontaneous or gaze induced. The physical examination is of great use in ruling out alternative diagnoses. Head thrust examination and head shake examination may induce nystagmus or augment spontaneous nystagmus. Tuning fork examination should also be performed to assess for asymmetry in hearing. In patients with labyrinthitis, the Weber examination is lateralized to the contralateral ear. However, the Rinne examination is positive (i.e., air conduction greater than bone conduction). In most cases, the remainder of the physical examination is unrevealing in labyrinthitis. The presence of additional neurologic findings on examination should prompt further evaluation and clinical suspicion of an alternative diagnosis.

The diagnostic evaluation of labyrinthitis may include audiometric evaluation, vestibular testing, and imaging of the temporal bone. Audiometric evaluation including pure tone audiometry, speech discrimination testing, tympanometry, and acoustic reflexes should be performed when patients present with complaints of hearing loss as in labyrinthitis. Pure tone audiometry may vary depending on the etiology of labyrinthitis. Because viral labyrinthitis is the most common form of labyrinthitis, audiometric evaluation most commonly reveals a mild to moderate high-frequency sensorineural hearing loss in the involved ear. However, a mixed loss with a conductive component may be identified, particularly in cases of suppurative labyrinthitis. Additionally, suppurative labyrinthitis is typically associated with a higher degree of hearing loss with a severe to profound sensorineural component. Tympanometry in these patients may reveal a flat response correlating with the presence of associated middle ear effusion. Patients with labyrinthitis in association with meningitis often present with bilateral hearing loss. Vestibular testing, including electronystagmography or videonystagmography, reveals a weakness in the involved ear, the ear with decreased hearing. Imaging including high-resolution computed tomography of the temporal bones or magnetic resonance imaging of the skull base can be of assistance in excluding disease processes within the differential. Computed tomography of the temporal bone is of particular assistance in diagnosis of mastoiditis as the etiology of labyrinthitis. Magnetic resonance imaging of the skull base in cases of labyrinthitis may reveal enhancement of the cochlea, vestibule, and semicircular canals on T1-weighted magnetic resonance imaging with gadolinium contrast.[5,6] The most common causes of vertigo are included in Figure 10-2 in the previous chapter. However, there is an extensive differential for labyrinthitis including but not limited to

- Brainstem hemorrhage
- Brainstem ischemia
- Cerebellar hemorrhage
- Cerebellar ischemia

- Ménière's disease
- Multiple sclerosis
- Ototoxin exposure
- Perilymphatic fistula/traumatic disruption of the otic capsule
- Presbystasis
- Tumors of the internal auditory canal, brainstem, or cerebellopontine angle
- Vestibular migraine
- Vertebral artery dissection
- Vertebrobasilar insufficiency
- Vestibular neuritis

TREATMENT

The treatment of labyrinthitis varies somewhat depending on the etiology of disease. In cases of suppurative labyrinthitis antibiotic therapy and operative management is indicated. Operative management may entail interventions ranging from myringotomy to mastoidectomy in cases of complicated otomastoiditis or cholesteatoma. Cultures should be obtained to guide antibiotic therapy. The mainstay of treatment for viral labyrinthitis is supportive including bedrest, hydration, and antiemetic medications. Vestibular suppressants are of benefit in reducing the severe symptoms of vertigo, but their use should be limited because they may compromise central vestibular compensation. Antiviral therapy and corticosteroid use in the treatment of labyrinthitis is controversial because there is no definitive evidence supporting their effect in improving outcomes. Vestibular therapy has been demonstrated to facilitate compensation in patients with long-term symptoms.[7]

> **KEY POINTS TO REMEMBER**
>
> - Labyrinthitis does have associated hearing loss
> - The etiology of labyrinthitis is most commonly viral, but bacterial and autoimmune etiology should be considered
> - Treatment is determined by etiology

Further Reading

1. Gulya AJ. Infections of the labyrinth. In: Bailey BJ, Johnson JT, Pillsbury HC, et al, editors. Head and Neck Surgery—Otolaryngology. Vol 2. Philadelphia: JB Lippincott, 1993. pp. 1769–81.
2. Jang CH, Park SY, Wang PC. A case of tympanogenic labyrinthitis complicated by acute otitis media. Yonsei Med J 2005;46:161–5.
3. Berlow SJ, Caldarelli DD, Matz GJ, et al. Bacterial meningitis and sensorineural hearing loss: a prospective investigation. Laryngoscope 1980;90:1445–52.
4. Rauch SD. Vestibular histopathology of the human temporal bone. What can we learn? Ann NY Acad Sci 2001;942:25–33.
5. Mark AS, Seltzer S, Nelson-Drake J, et al. Labyrinthine enhancement of gadolinium-enhanced magnetic resonance imaging in sudden deafness and vertigo: correlation with audiologic and electronystagmographic studies. Ann Otol Rhinol Laryngol 1992;101:459–64.
6. Kopelovich JC, Germiller JA, Laury AM, et al. Early prediction of postmeningitic hearing loss in children using magnetic resonance imaging. Arch Otolaryngol Head Neck Surg 2011;137:441–7.
7. Cohen HS, Kimball KT. Decreased ataxia and improved balance after vestibular rehabilitation. Otolaryngol Head Neck Surg 2004;130:418–25.

12 Benign Paroxysmal Positional Vertigo

A 52-year-old female presents for evaluation of vertigo. She states that vertigo began approximately 2 weeks ago following an accident in which she struck her head while attempting to enter a car. She describes episodes of true horizontal axis vertigo lasting approximately 20 seconds on average. The episodes of vertigo resolve spontaneously. She notes an association with certain head movements. She denies nausea or emesis. There is no hearing loss, tinnitus, aural fullness, otalgia, otorrhea, or previous incidents of vertigo prior to 2 weeks ago. Her past medical history is significant for type 2 diabetes mellitus. Her past surgical history is significant for cholecystectomy. She has no other significant trauma history. Medications include metformin and a daily multivitamin. Social history is unremarkable. Physical examination reveals her Weber to be midline and Rinne to be positive (air conduction greater than bone conduction bilaterally). The otologic examination is unremarkable. The neurologic examination is within normal limits as is the remainder of the head and neck examination. The Dix-Hallpike maneuver was performed and found to be positive on the right.

What do you do now?

Benign paroxysmal positional vertigo (BPPV) is the most common cause of vertigo in the United States. Most cases of BPPV are idiopathic followed in frequency by those associated with head trauma. However, BPPV may occur as a concomitant disease process in association with other forms of vertigo or otologic disease (i.e., Ménière's disease or vestibular neuronitis). The pathophysiology of BPPV is postulated to be secondary to either canalithiasis or cupulolithiasis. With regard to canalithiasis, otoconia are thought to be mobile and free floating within the semicircular canals; vertigo result from exertion of force by the otoconia within the semicircular canals. With regard to cupulolithiasis, densities caused by adherent otoconia to the cupula of the crista ampullaris result in the presentation of vertigo.

The annual incidence of BPPV is believed to range from 10 to 60 per 100,000 population with an overall prevalence of 2.4%.[1-3] A female preponderance has been noted. As such, the female prevalence has been reported as 3.2% versus a male prevalence of 1.6%.[3] BPPV is most common among individuals between the ages of 50 and 70 years, but can occur at any age.[4] In younger patients, a history of recent head trauma is often associated.

BPPV is classified according to the semicircular canal involved. Most cases of BPPV involve the posterior semicircular canal. Approximately, 90%–95% of cases of BPPV are attributed to posterior canal BPPV.[5] Horizontal canal BPPV is the second most common form of BPPV accounting for approximately 5%–15% of cases.[6,7] Because posterior canal BPPV accounts for most cases, the remainder of this chapter is focused on posterior canal disease.

The clinical presentation of BPPV is typically one of sudden onset. Patients tend to present with symptoms of vertigo with a positional association. Patients often complain of dizziness or vertigo when going into the supine position with the affected ear down. The vertigo typically lasts 15–30 seconds. The intensity of the vertigo may vary from individual to individual. Some patients report a feeling of fogginess or cloudiness at baseline in association with BPPV. As with other forms of vertigo obtaining a detailed history of present illness is critical because BPPV diagnosis is largely based on reported symptomatology.

On physical examination, the otologic examination is typically normal. Similarly, the neurologic examination typically does not reveal significant findings. The head and neck examination is also typically unrevealing. The Dix-Hallpike test is of assistance in confirming the diagnosis of BPPV. During the Dix-Hallpike test, the patient's head is turned 45 degrees to one side while sitting upright. The patient is then reclined to the supine position with the head position at a 30-degree angle below the plane of the floor (Figure 12-1).[8] If the test is positive, a brief latency of a few seconds is observed followed by rotatory nystagmus when the affected ear is down. This nystagmus lasts approximately 15–30 seconds. The patient similarly reports sensation of vertigo with onset of nystagmus. If the horizontal canal is involved, the nystagmus may be horizontal axis instead of rotatory. Nystagmus and vertigo may be elicited on sitting the patient upright again. With BPPV, this response tends to be fatigable.

The options for treatment of BPPV include vestibular suppressants, canalith repositioning, vestibular therapy, or surgical management. Of these modalities, canalith reposition is most commonly used and has been found to have the greatest success in resolution of symptoms. Figure 12-2 presents the Epley maneuver, a common canalith reposition technique used for posterior BPPV.[9] Alternatively for horizontal BPPV the Lempert 360-degree supine roll maneuver may be used. Occasionally,

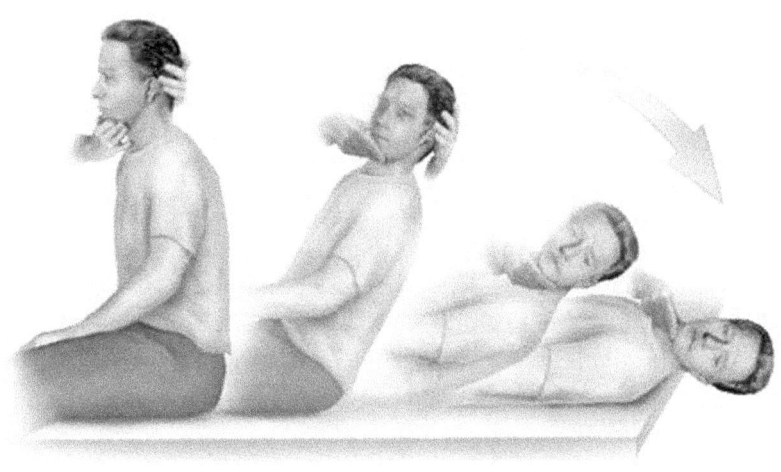

FIGURE 12-1 Illustration of the Dix-Hallpike maneuver. Source: http://www.medicinageriatrica.com.br/2007/05/09/manobra-de-dix-hallpike./ Date Accessed: January 21, 2013

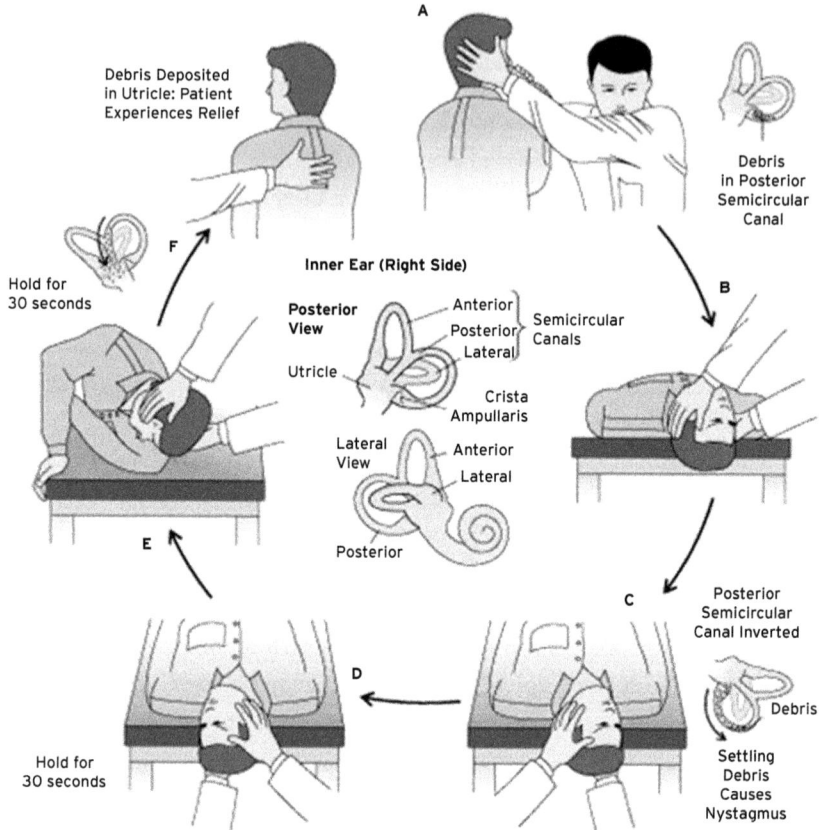

FIGURE 12-2 Illustration of Epley maneuver. Source: http://www.drpaulose.com/ear/ent-pediatric-children/positional-vertigo-get-medical-help. Date Accessed: January 21, 2013

patients may require more than one episode of treatment for resolution of symptoms. It has been reported that 78% of patients experience resolution of symptoms with one canalith repositioning treatment.[10] The success rate increases to 90% with two canalith repositioning treatments.[10,11] Vestibular therapy similarly is of benefit in providing patients with exercises that emphasize compensation and habituation.[12] In most patients canalith repositioning treatment and vestibular therapy are sufficient to alleviate disease. However, in a select minority of patients severe symptoms persist, necessitating operative management. Although singular nerve sectioning has previously been reported in the literature, the most common operative procedure used for recalcitrant BPPV is selective canal plugging. This is rarely required because most patients with vestibular therapy or repositioning maneuvers are able to habituate to the associated changes.

The recurrence rate of BPPV is quite high. In most studies, a recurrence rate of approximately 15% per year has been reported.[11,13,14] The management of recurrent episodes similarly includes canalith repositioning and vestibular therapy as first-line treatments.

KEY POINTS TO REMEMBER

- BPPV is the most common cause of vertigo
- Symptoms typically last seconds
- Canalith repositioning is typically successful in relief of symptoms
- The recurrence rate is approximately 15%

Further Reading

1. Mizukoshi K, Watanabe Y, Shojaku H, et al. Epidemiological studies on benign paroxysmal positional vertigo in Japan. Acta Otolaryngol Suppl 1998;447:67–72.
2. Froehling DA, Silverstein MD, Mohr DN, et al. Benign positional vertigo: incidence and prognosis in a population-based study in Olmsted County, Minnesota. Mayo Clin Proc 1991;66:596–601.
3. Von Brevern M, Radtke A, Lezius F, et al. Epidemiology of benign paroxysmal positional vertigo: a population based study. J Neurol Neurosurg Psychiatry 2007;78:710–5.
4. Baloh RW, Honrubia V, Jacobson K. Benign positional vertigo: clinical and oculographic features in 240 cases. Neurology 1987;37:371–8.
5. Honrubia V, Baloh RW, Harris MR, et al. Paroxysmal positional vertigo syndrome. Am J Otol 1999;20:465–70.
6. Cakir BO, Ercan I, Cakir ZA, et al. What is the true incidence of horizontal semicircular canal benign paroxysmal positional vertigo? Otolaryngol Head Neck Surg 2006;134:451–4.
7. Parnes LS, Agrawal SK, Atlas J. Diagnosis and management of benign paroxysmal positional vertigo (BPPV). CMAJ 2003;169:681–93.
8. <http://www.medicinageriatrica.com.br/2007/05/09/manobra-de-dix-hallpike/>. Date Accessed: January 21, 2013.
9. <http://www.drpaulose.com/ear/ent-pediatric-children/positional-vertigo-get-medical-help>. Date Accessed: January 21, 2013.

10. White J, Savvides P, Cherian N, et al. Canalith repositioning for benign parozysmal positional vertigo. Otol Neurotol 2005;26:704–10.
11. Nunez RA, Cass SP, Furman JM. Short- and long-term outcomes of canalith repositioning for benign paroxysmal positional vertigo. Otolaryngol Head Neck Surg 2000;122:647–52.
12. Brandt T, Daroff RB. Physical therapy for benign paroxysmal positional vertigo. Arch Otolaryngol 1980;106:484–5.
13. Epley JM. The canalith repositioning procedure: for treatment of benign paroxysmal positional vertigo. Otolaryngol Head Neck Surg 1992;107:399–404.
14. Furman JM, Cass SP. Benign paroxysmal positional vertigo. N Engl J Med 1999;341:1590–6.

13 Migrainous Vertigo

A 37-year-old female presents for evaluation of vertigo. She states that she has three to five episodes per month. This started approximately 1 year ago. She describes episodes lasting 30 minutes to half a day. She has noted right temporal headache with some episodes of vertigo. She denies associated hearing loss, preceding tinnitus, or aural pressure. She has on occasion "bright spots" in her visual field prior to onset of vertigo. The sensation of vertigo during episodes ranges from true horizontal axis vertigo to feeling of the "ground moving like waves in the ocean" or "the world swaying." She inconsistently experiences nausea and emesis with these episodes. She describes photophobia and phonophobia in association with and prior to these episodes. Her past medical history is significant for migraine headaches particularly during menses for which she symptomatically takes over-the-counter migraine medications. There is no past surgical or trauma history. She denies tobacco or recreational drug use. She consumes one to two glasses of only white wine weekly, because red wine causes headaches. She consumes two to three cups of caffeinated beverages daily. Physical examination is unremarkable.

What do you do now?

Migrainous vertigo is relatively common. The overall prevalence of migraine within the population is approximately 10%.[1] Among patients with a history of migraine, dizziness or vertigo has been reported in 3%–9% of the population.[2-5] As such, the overall prevalence of migrainous vertigo in the general population has been estimated to be approximately 1%, making migrainous vertigo 5–10 times more common than Ménière's disease.[6-8] Migrainous vertigo is three times more prevalent within the female population and has been noted to have a high rate of association with other otologic diseases.[8,9]

Currently, there is no gold standard or universally recognized diagnostic criteria for migrainous vertigo.[8,10] Various diagnostic criteria systems have been proposed within the literature.[11,12] The most commonly used and advocated diagnostic criteria were proposed by Neuhauser and colleagues in 2001.[3,8,10] Neuhauser et al.[3] describe the diagnosis of vestibular migraine as definite or probable, defining them respectively as follows:

Definite vestibular migraine
- Episodic vestibular symptoms of at least moderate severity
- Current or previous history of migraine according to the *International Classification of Headache Disorders 2nd Edition*[13] or migrainous symptoms during two or more attacks of vertigo (migrainous headache, photophobia, phonophobia, visual aura or other aura)
- Other causes ruled out by appropriate investigation

Probable vestibular migraine
- Episodic vestibular symptoms of at least moderate severity
- One of the following:
  - Current or previous history of migraine according to the *International Classification of Headache Disorders 2nd Edition*
  - Migrainous symptoms during vestibular symptoms
  - Migraine precipitants of vertigo in more that 50% of attacks (food triggers, sleep irregularities, or hormonal change)
  - Response to migraine medications in more than 50% of attacks.
- Other causes ruled out by appropriate investigations.

In a validation study of the criteria designated by Neuhauser et al.,[3] half of all patients with an initial diagnosis of probable migrainous vertigo later went on to be reclassified as definite migrainous vertigo at a mean follow-up of approximately 8 years.[14] Thirty-two percent of patients maintained a diagnosis of probable migrainous vertigo, whereas the remainder of patients attained alternative diagnoses including Ménière's disease.[14]

The pathophysiology of migrainous vertigo is believed to be one of hyperexcitability to various forms of external stimuli (i.e., bright light, loud sounds, smells, and motion) both during migraine episodes and at baseline.[15,16] It has been theorized that migraine aura represents vasoconstriction and cortical hypoxia in conjunction with a cortical neuronal process involving the trigeminal brainstem circuitry.[17-22] Thickening of the sensory cortex has also been described.[23]

The diagnosis of migrainous vertigo is largely a diagnosis of exclusion. As such, alternative diagnoses should be excluded in the diagnostic evaluation. The differential diagnosis of headache with vertigo includes but is not limited to posttraumatic vertigo, vertebrobasilar insufficiency or thrombosis, Ménière's disease, internal auditory canal or cerebellopontine angle tumors, familial episodic ataxia, cyclic vomiting syndrome, benign paroxysmal positional vertigo, temporal bone malignancy, basilar meningitis, and temporal lobe epilepsy.

CLINICAL PRESENTATION

As with traditional migraine, migrainous vertigo is commonly associated with aura. In the study by Radtke et al.,[14] 63% of patients with definite migrainous vertigo and 22% of probable migrainous vertigo reported aura in association with episodes. The onset of symptoms may present as gradual or abrupt. In most cases the duration of symptoms ranges from 5 to 60 minutes; however, symptoms lasting from seconds to greater than 24 hours have been described.[3] Headache is not always associated with symptoms of vertigo. Approximately 45% of patients report headache consistently with vertigo, approximately 48% report headache sometimes with vertigo, and approximately 6% report never experiencing headache with vertigo.[3]

The most common symptoms reported in association with migrainous vertigo are rotational vertigo, intolerance of head motion, and positional vertigo reported in 70%, 48%, and 42% of patients, respectively.[3] Other symptoms reported include intolerance to visual motion, motion sickness, sensation of floating, rocking, tilting, walking on an uneven surface,

TABLE 13-1 **Triggers for Migrainous Vertigo**

Category	Triggers
Weather	Storm fronts
	Rapid changes in barometric pressure
	Change of season
Environmental	Strong smells or perfumes
	Bright lights (fluorescent lights)
	Tight spaces (crowds)
	Visualization of motion (watching trains pass)
Activity	Physical exertion
	Dehydration
	Sleep deprivation
Hormonal	Menses
Dietary	Caffeine (intake or change in intake pattern)
	Chocolate
	Alcohol
	Aged cheese
	Monosodium glutamate
	Nitrites

unsteadiness, balance disturbance, and lightheadedness.[8,12] Photophobia, phonophobia, and auras other than vertigo are commonly associated.[3] As with traditional migraine, triggers have been described. Common triggers are presented in Table 13-1.[8,12] Latency may present between exposure to the trigger and onset of symptoms. Although rare, episodic hearing loss has also been described in cases of migrainous vertigo.[24-27]

DIAGNOSTIC EVALUATION

The diagnosis of migrainous vertigo is largely a diagnosis of exclusion based mainly on clinical history. The diagnostic evaluation of patients with headache and vertigo should begin with a physical examination including a complete neurologic and head and neck examination. In patients with migrainous vertigo, the examination is typically normal. However, patients may present with nystagmus during acute attacks that is only discernible with video Frenzel goggle examination.[28,29]

No confirmatory tests currently exist to definitively establish the diagnosis of migrainous vertigo. Therefore, additional testing in patients with presumed migrainous vertigo is focused on excluding alternative diagnoses. A formal audiometric evaluation may be performed to assess for asymmetric sensorineural hearing loss in association with symptoms. Electronystagmography, videonystagmography, or vestibular evoked myogenic potentials may be performed to assess for peripheral vestibular hypofunction. Magnetic resonance imaging of the temporal bone and posterior fossa may be performed to exclude central lesions as the etiology for symptoms. Less commonly rotational chair or posturography may be performed.

NATURAL HISTORY

To date, no studies have specifically explored the natural history of migrainous vertigo. However, if the natural history of migrainous vertigo parallels that of traditional migraines, one may expect symptoms to worsen during the childbearing years and decrease in frequency and severity after menopause.

TREATMENT

Patients should be encouraged to maintain a detailed dietary and activity log to identify potential triggers for possible elimination. Treatment of migraine symptoms has been demonstrated to alleviate dizziness and vertigo in most cases.[30] Multiple studies have evaluated the potential of various medical therapies as prophylaxis for migrainous vertigo; however, few represent level I evidence.[31] However, among these studies, positive results with prophylactic therapy have been demonstrated at decreasing symptom frequency and severity. Agents that have been described for prophylaxis in migrainous vertigo include

- Carbonic anhydrase-inhibitors acetazolamide[32]
- Dichlorphenamid[33]
- Flunarizine[34]
- Lamotrigine[35]
- Metoprolol[34]
- Pizotifen[30,36]
- Propranolol[37]
- Topiramate[38]
- Tricyclic antidepressants[30]

Additionally, abortive therapies including triptans and vestibular suppressants have been demonstrated to be beneficial in alleviating symptoms of headache and vertigo during acute migraine attacks.[39-41]

> **KEY POINTS TO REMEMBER**
>
> - Migraine-associated vertigo is often described as "boat-like vertigo" or swaying motion
> - Photophobia and/or phonophobia is often associated
> - Migraine-associated vertigo is 5-10 times more common than Ménière's disease
> - Treatment entails standard migraine medications

Further Reading

1. Stewart W, Shechter A, Rasmussen B. Migraine prevalence. A review of population based studies. Neurology 1994;44:S17-23.
2. Selby G, Lancer JW. Observations on 500 cases of migraine and allied vascular headache. J Neurol Neurosurg Psychiatry 1960;23:23-32.
3. Neuhauser H, Leopold M, von Brevern M, et al. The interactions of migraine, vertigo, and migrainous vertigo. Neurology 2001;56:436-41.
4. Lempert T, Neuhauser H. Epidemiology of vertigo, migraine and vestibular migraine. J Neurol 2009;256:333-8.
5. Neuhauser H, von Brevern M, Radtke A, et al. Epidemiology of vestibular vertigo: a neurotologic survey of the general population. Neurology 2005;65:898-904.
6. Neuhauser H, Lempert T. Vestibular migraine. Neurol Clin 2009;27:379-91.
7. Neuhauser H, Radtke A, von Brevern M, et al. Migrainous vertigo: prevalence and impact on quality of life. Neurology 2006;67:1028-33.
8. Cherchi M, Hain TC. Migraine-associated vertigo. Otolaryngol Clin North Am 2011;44:367-75.

9. Lipton RB, Bigal ME, Diamond M, et al. Migraine prevalence, disease burden, and the need for preventive therapy. Neurology 2007;68:343–9.
10. Kahmke R, Kaylie D. What are the diagnostic criteria for migraine-associated vertigo? Laryngoscope 2012;122:1885–6.
11. Brantberg K, Trees N, Baloh RW. Migraine-associated vertigo. Acta Otolaryngol 2005;125:276–9.
12. Cohen JM, Bigal ME, Newman LC. Migraine and vestibular symptoms-identifying clinical features that predict "vestibular migraine." Headache 2011;51:1393–7.
13. Headache Classification Subcommittee of the International Headache Society. The international classification of headache disorders: 2nd edition. Cephalalgia 2004;24:9–160.
14. Radtke A, Neuhauser H, von Brevern M, et al. Vestibular migraine-validity of clinical diagnostic criteria. Cephalalgia 2011;31:906–13.
15. Aurora SK, Wilkinson F. The brain is hyperexcitable in migraine. Cephalalgia 2007;27:1442–53.
16. Burstein R, Yarnitsky D, Goor-Aryeh I, et al. An association between migraine and cutaneous allodynia. Ann Neurol 2000;47:614–24.
17. Schreiber CP. The pathophysiology of migraine. Dis Mon 2006;52:385–401.
18. Leao AAP. Spreading depression of activity in the cerebral cortex. J Neurophysiol 1944;7:359–90.
19. Leao AAP, Morison RS. Propagation of spreading cortical depression. J Neurophysiol 1945;8:33–46.
20. Olesen J, Friber L, Olsen TS, et al. Timing and topography of cerebral blood flow, aura, and headache during migraine attacks. Ann Neurol 1990;28:791–8.
21. Welch KM. Concepts of migraine headache pathogenesis: insights into mechanisms of chronicity and new drug targets. Neurol Sci 2003;24:S149–53.
22. Ramadan NM. Targeting therapy for migraine: what to treat? Neurology 2005;64:S4–823.
23. DaSilva AF, Granziera C, Snyder J, et al. Thickening in the somatosensory cortex of patients with migraine. Neurology 2007;69:1990–5.
24. Lee H, Lopez I, Ishiyama A, et al. Can Migraine damage the inner ear? Arch Neurol 2000;57:1631–4.
25. Lee H, Whitman GT, Lim JG, et al. Hearing symptoms in migrainous infarction. Arch Neurol 2003;60:113–6.
26. Lipkin AF, Jenkins HA, Coker NJ. Migraine and sudden sensorineural hearing loss. Arch Otolaryngol Head Neck Surg 1987;113:325–6.
27. Viirre ES, Baloh RW. Migraine as a cause of sudden hearing loss. Headache 1996;36:24–8.
28. von Brevern M, Zeise D, Neuhauser H, et al. Acute migrainous vertigo: clinical and oculographic findings. Brain 2005;128:365–74.
29. Polensek SH, Tusa RJ. Nystagmus during attacks of vestibular migraine: an aid in diagnosis. Audiol Neurootol 2010;15:241–6.

30. Reploeg MD, Goebel JA. Migraine-associated dizziness: patient characteristics and management options. Otol Neurotol 2002;23:364–71.
31. Fotuhi M, Glaun B, Quan SY, et al. Vestibular migraine: a critical review of treatment trials. J Neurol 2009;256:711–6.
32. Baloh RW, Foster CA, Yue Q, Nelson SF, et al. Familial migraine with vertigo and essential tremor. Neurology 1996;46:458–60.
33. Asprella Libonati G, Gagliardi G. La malattia di Meniere e vertigine emicranica: terapia intercritica, terapia medica. Otoneurologia 2004;18:40–2.
34. Dieterich M, Brandt T. Episodic vertigo related to migraine (90 cases): vestibular migraine? J Neurol 1999;246:883–92.
35. Bisdorff AR. Treatment of migraine related vertigo with lamotrigine an observational study. Bull Soc Sci Med Grand Duche Luxemb 2004;2:103–8.
36. Waterson J. Chronic migrainous vertigo. J Clin Neurosci 2004;11:384–8.
37. Harker LA, Rassekh C. Migraine equivalent as a cause of episodic vertigo. Laryngoscope 1988;98:160–4.
38. Carmona S, Settecase N. Use of topiramate (topomax) in a subgroup of migraine-vertigo patients with auditory symptoms. Ann N Y Acad Sci 2005;1039:517–20.
39. Neuhauser H, Radtke A, von Brevern M, Lempert T, et al. Zolmitriptan for treatment of migrainous vertigo: a pilot randomized placebo-controlled trial. Neurology 2003;60:882–3.
40. Baloh RW. Neurotology of migraine. Headache 1997;37:615–21.
41. Bikhazi P, Jackson C, Ruckenstein MJ. Efficacy of antimigrainous therapy in the treatment of migraine-associated dizziness. Am J Otol 1997;18:350–4.

14 Perilymphatic Fistula

A 10-year-old male presents with his mother for evaluation of vertigo. He states that vertigo has been present for the past 10 days. The vertigo is exacerbated by straining and lifting. Of note, he was seen in the emergency department 10 days ago following a sledding accident. The patient fell off of his sled while sliding down a hill and was impaled in the right ear with a twig from a pine tree. He noted onset of vertigo on removal of the twig. He was taken to the emergency department for evaluation by his mother where he was noted to have a perforation of the tympanic membrane. No additional injuries were noted. He was discharged from the emergency department with instructions to follow-up with a specialist. He reports hearing loss on the right since the time of the accident. He has no history of otologic infections or surgeries. His past medical history is significant for attention-deficit/hyperactivity disorder. On physical examination, the patient is a well-nourished 10-year-old male. On otoscopy, the patient was noted to have mild scarring from a spontaneous repair of the tympanic membrane perforation. Vertigo was reported and nystagmus was inducible on pneumatic otoscopy of the right ear. The head and neck examination was within normal limits. Neurologic examination revealed positive tandem walking and Romberg tests. Audiometric evaluation revealed a mild-to-moderate left sensorineural hearing loss (Figure 14-1). High-resolution computed tomography (CT) of the temporal bones revealed subluxation of the stapes and moderate pneumolabyrinth.

What do you do now?

The patient in this case exhibits findings consistent with a diagnosis of traumatic perilymphatic fistula. A perilymphatic fistula is abnormal communication between the perilymphatic space of the inner ear with the middle ear or mastoid. The leakage of perilyph out of the perilymphatic spaces in the inner ear leads to an imbalance in the perilymph to endolymph ratio precipitating symptoms of hearing loss and vertigo. The incidence and prevalence of perilymphatic fistula is unknown. Perilymphatic fistulas may occur as a function of trauma, iatrogenic injury (following otologic surgery, such as stapedectomy or cochlear implantation), congenital anomalies, or idiopathic/spontaneous etiologies secondary to hydrodynamic forces.

Two mechanisms of injury pertaining to hydrodynamic forces have been proposed classically by Goodhill and Ben[1] in 1981: explosive injury and implosive injury. Explosive injury results from increases in intracranial pressure and cerebrospinal fluid pressure levels, which is transmitted to the perilymphatic space via the cochlear aqueduct or lamina cribosa. This can occur from strain, coughing, or sneezing leading to tears in the oval window annulus or round window membrane. Implosive injury results

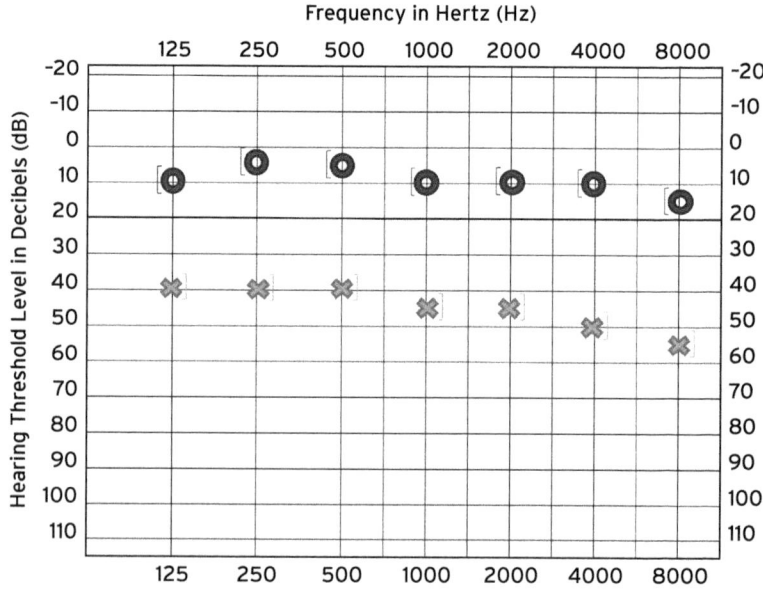

FIGURE 14-1 Pure tone audiogram from patient with vertigo following penetrating ear trauma.

from severe excursion of the tympanic membrane, acoustic trauma, or direct positive pressure on the oval or round window, such as in sudden decompression syndrome in scuba diving. In scuba injuries, round window rupture has most commonly been reported.[2] Interestingly, flight attendant travel with acute upper respiratory tract infections has been associated with an increased risk of perilymphatic fistula development.[3] The most common etiologic factor in the development of perilymphatic fistula is trauma.[4-6] Various foreign bodies have been reported in the literature as the traumatic cause of perilymphatic fistula including knitting needles, hairpins, bullets, twigs from a tree, ear picks, cotton-tipped applicators, and stones.[7-15]

The clinical presentation of perilymphatic fistula overlaps greatly with other vestibular disorders making it somewhat challenging to diagnose. Obtaining a detailed history of present illness is of critical importance. Patients with perilymphatic fistulas most commonly present with hearing loss and vertigo, but may also present with complaints of tinnitus, aural fullness, disequilibrium, or motion intolerance.[16-18] These symptoms may vary in severity and complexity ranging from mild symptoms to incapacitating disease. Hearing loss in association with perilymphatic fistula may present as sudden onset or fluctuating. Patients may present with hearing loss ranging from mild to profound hearing loss. A positive Tullio phenomenon may also be reported.

On physical examination, otoscopy may reveal a normal tympanic membrane or signs consistent with previous penetrating trauma. Spontaneous nystagmus is rare. A fistula test should be performed with the pneumatic otoscope by applying positive pressure to the tympanic membrane. Objective observation of induced nystagmus or subjective onset of vertigo or dysequilibrium signifies a positive fistula test. However, a positive fistula test correlates with an actual fistula in only 24%–77% of case.[16] Patients may present with a positive tandem Romberg test.

Audiometric evaluation should be performed. Sensorineural hearing loss is most commonly encountered; however, patients may present with a mixed loss. Dynamic platform posturography testing may be positive for dysequilibrium with a vestibular pattern or swaying with positive pressure applied to the tympanic membrane. Electronysgamography or videonystagmostraphy may reveal a unilateral asymmetric weakness on the involved side. An elevated summation potential to action potential ratio on

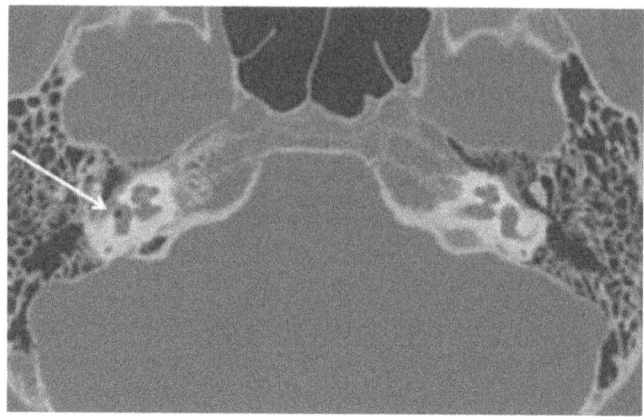

FIGURE 14-2 Axial CT scan demonstrating pneumolabyrinth (*arrow*). Source: Reproduced with the permission of Khoo LS, Tan TY. Traumatic perilymphatic fistula secondary to stapes luxation into the vestibule: a case report. ENT Journal 2011;90:E29-E31.

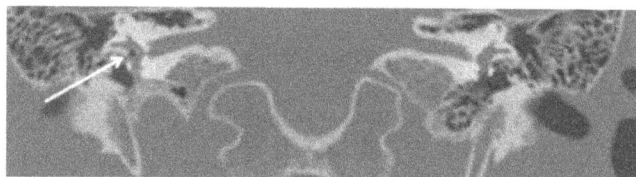

FIGURE 14-3 Coronal CT scan demonstrating pneumolabyrinth (*arrow*). Source: Reproduced with the permission of Khoo LS, Tan TY. Traumatic perilymphatic fistula secondary to stapes luxation into the vestibule: a case report. ENT Journal 2011;90:E29-E31.

electrocochleography raises the clinical suspicion of perilymphatic fistula. It is important to note that the summation potential to action potential ratio may also be elevated in Ménière's disease, which has a similar clinical presentation.

Imaging of the temporal bone may be of benefit in confirming the diagnosis. However, lack of findings does not preclude the diagnosis of perilymphatic fistula. Pneumolabyrinth on high-resolution CT of the temporal bone increases the clinical suspicion for perilymphatic fistula (Figure 14-2 and Figure 14-3).[19] Additionally, subluxation of the stapes or ossicular anomalies may be visualized on high-resolution CT of the temporal bone in cases of potential traumatic perilymphatic fistula. Without a definitive history of an inciting incident and because of the similarity in presenting symptoms, magnetic resonance imaging of the posterior fossa may be obtained to rule out tumors involving the internal auditory canal or cerebellopontine angle.

The treatment of perilymphatic fistula remains controversial. For nontraumatic or idiopathic perilymphatic fistulas, conservative management including bed rest, elevation of the head of the bed, stool softeners, and avoidance of increase in intracranial pressure may be used initially with surgical exploration only performed for failures of conservative management. Alternatively, certain surgeons advocate exploration in all patients with a suspicion for perilymphatic fistula. There are no absolute contraindications for surgical exploration. However, exploration should be embarked on judiciously in patients with unilateral deafness when considering exploration in the only hearing ear. Exploration may be performed under general anesthesia or under local anesthesia with mild sedation.

During the exploration procedure, the tympanic membrane is elevated allowing for visualization of the middle ear contents including the oval and round window for assessment of active perilymphatic leakage. Intrathecal fluorescein may be used to assist in the identification of the site of leak. However, because of the low sensitivity and risks involved in intrathecal fluorescein administration, its use is not advocated by most surgeons.[20] Alternatively, cochlin-tomoprotein has been investigated as a tool to assist in the identification of active perilymphatic leakage. Cochlin-tomoprotein tests positive by Western blot assay in all perilymph samples and negative in greater than 98% of nonperilyph samples lending to high test sensitivity and specificity.[21,22] However, cochlin-tomoprotein testing is not routinely available, and its use remains largely experimental.

Regardless of the visualization of active leakage, repair is often used in all patients who undergo exploration because repair does not result in a significant risk of postoperative hearing loss and often prevents further hearing loss even when fistula is not identified intraoperatively.[23] A fascia patch is most commonly used to occlude the round window and oval window.[24] However, limited studies have revealed autologous blood patches to be of promise in perilymphatic fistula repair.[25]

Exploration and repair in the management of perilymphatic fistula has been found to be highly effective for vestibular symptoms but less so for hearing loss. Approximately 80%–95% of patients experience improvement in vestibular function following perilymphatic fistula repair.[17,26,27]

Conversely, variable results have been reported with regard to improvement in hearing following perilymphatic fistula repair ranging from approximately 10%–50% with significantly lower rates of serviceable hearing.[17,26,27] Perilymphatic fistula repair, however, is more successful in stabilization of hearing in most patients.[17,26-28]

KEY POINTS TO REMEMBER

- The etiology of perilymphatic fistula is most commonly trauma or iatrogenic; however, congenital and spontaneous etiologies have been described
- Vertigo and hearing loss are commonly associated
- Assessment for a positive Tullio phenomenon should be performed
- Treatment remains controversial

Further Reading
1. Goodhill V, Ben H. Senturia lecture. Leaking labyrinth lesions, deafness, tinnitus and dizziness. Ann Otol Rhinol Laryngol 1981;90:99–106.
2. Pullen FW II. Perilymphatic fistula induced by barotrauma. Am J Otol 1992;13:270–2.
3. Klokker M, Vesterhauge S. Perilymphatic fistula in cabin attendants: an incapacitating consequence of flying with common cold. Aviat Space Environ Med 2005;76:66–8.
4. Strohm M. Traumatic lesions of the round window membrane and perilymphatic fistulae. Adv Otol Rhinol Laryngol 1986;35:177–247.
5. Fitzgerald DC. Head trauma: hearing loss and dizziness. J Trauma 1996;40:488–96.
6. Grimm RG, Hemenway WG, LeBray PR, Black FO, et al. The perilyph fistula syndrome defined in mild head trauma. Acta Otolaryngol 1989;64:5–40.
7. Kobayashi T, Gyo K. Earpick injury of the stapes. Am J Otolaryngol 2000;21:340–3.
8. Vanderstock L, Varmeersch H, DeVel E. Traumatic luxation of the stapes. J Laryngol Otol 1983;97:533–7.
9. Herman P, Guichard JP, Van den Abbeele T, et al. Traumatic luxation of the stapes evidence by high-resolution CT. AJNR Am J Neuroradiol 1996;17:1242–4.
10. Yamasoba T, Amagai N, Karino S. Traumatic luxation of the stapes into the vestibule. Otolaryngol Head Neck Surg 2003;129:287–90.
11. Lao WW, Niparko JK. Assessment of changes in cochlear function with pneumolabyrinth after middle ear trauma. Otol Neurotol 2007;28:1013–17
12. Hatano A, Rikitake M, Komori M, et al. Traumatic perilymphatic fistula with the luxation of the stapes into the vestibule. Auris Nasus Larynx 2009;36:474–8.

13. Snelling JD, Bennett A, Wilson P, Wickstead M, et al. Unusual middle-ear mischief: trans-tympanic trauma from a hair grip resulting in ossicular, facial nerve and oval window disruption. J Laryngol Otol 2006;120:793–5.
14. Ederies A, Yuen HW, Chen JW, et al. Traumatic stapes fracture with rotation and subluxation into the vestibule and pneumolabyrinth. Laryngoscope 2009;119:1195–7.
15. Meriot P, Veillon F, Garcia JF, et al. CT appearance of ossicular injury. Radiographics 1997;17:1445–54.
16. Kveton JF. Perilymph fistulae. In: Pensak ML, editor. Controversies in Otolaryngology. New York: Theime Medical Publishers, Inc., 2001. pp. 303–6.
17. Seltzer S, McCabe BF. Perilymph fistula: the Iowa experience. Laryngoscope 1986;96:37–49.
18. Glasscick ME III, Hart MJ, Rosdeutscher JD, et al. Traumatic perilymphatic fistula: how long can symptoms persist? A follow-up report. Am J Otol 1992;13:333–8.
19. Khoo LS, Tan TY. Traumatic perilymphatic fistula secondary to stapes luxation into the vestibule: a case report. ENT Journal 2011;90:E28-E31.
20. Gehrking E, Wisst F, Remmert S, Sommer K, et al. Intraoperative assessment of perilymphatic fistulas with intrathecal administration of fluorescein. Laryngoscope 2002;112:1614–8.
21. Ikezono T, Shindo Sekine K, et al. Cochlin-tomoprotein (CTP) detection test identifies traumatic perilymphatic fistula due to penetrating middle ear injury. Acta Otolaryngol 2011;131:937–44.
22. Ikezono T, Shindo, Sekiguchi S, et al. The performance of cochlin-tomoprotein detection testing the diagnosis of perilymphatic fistula. Audiol Neurootol 2010;15:168–74.
23. Weber PC, Bluestone CD, Perez B. Outcome of hearing and vertigo after surgery for congenital perilymphatic fistula in children. Am J Otolaryngol 2003;24:138–42.
24. Emmett JR, Shea JJ. Traumatic perilymph fistula. Laryngoscope 1980;90:1513–20.
25. Garg R, Djalilian HR. Intratympanic injection of autologous blood for traumatic perilymphatic fistulas. Otolaryngol Head Neck Surg 2009;141:294–5.
26. Black FO, Pesznecker S, Norton T, et al. Surgical management of perilymphatic fistulas: a Portland experience. Am J Otol 1992;13:254–62.
27. Rizer FM. House JW. Perilymph fistulas: the House Ear Clinic experience. Otolaryngol Head Neck Surg 1991;104:239–43.
28. Weber PC, Bluestone CD, Perez B. Surgical outcome of perilymphatic fistula surgery. Paper presented at: the Annual Meeting of the American Otological, Rhinological and Laryngological Society; April 1993; Los Angeles, CA.

15 Superior Semicircular Canal Dehiscence

A 37-year-old female presents for evaluation of vertigo. She states that the problem began almost immediately following minor trauma in which she was accidentally hit in the chin by her son's forehead while playing basketball 3 months ago. She did not sustain any facial or mandible fractures per computed tomography (CT) performed by her primary care provider on evaluation. She states that discomfort from the accident abated after approximately 1 week, but she still experiences a myriad of symptoms including right autophony, hearing her own heartbeat, and hearing her footsteps in her right ear when jogging. She reports dizziness or sensation of "the world moving like an arc" with nose blowing, while vacuuming, when her children are playing loudly, and during bowel movements. She denies associated nausea or emesis. There is no tinnitus or hearing loss. Past medical history is unremarkable. She takes no medications. Physical examination revealed no gaze nystagmus and a negative Dix-Hallpike. On tuning fork examination, the Weber lateralized to the right. The otologic examination was within normal limits with the exception of up-beating nystagmus elicited on pneumatic otoscopy. The remainder of the neurologic, head, and neck examination was within normal limits. The audiogram obtained revealed a borderline right air-bone gap at the low frequencies (Figure 15-1). High-resolution CT of the temporal bones was obtained, which revealed dehiscence of the bone overlying the superior semicircular canal (Figure 15-2).

What do you do now?

Semicircular canal dehiscence represents an abnormal communication between the inner ear and surrounding structure through a lack of an osseous covering over the membranous labyrinth. This creates a third window in the inner ear, disrupting its normal mechanism, causing characteristic symptoms of vertigo and/or hearing loss.[1] Dehiscence in all semicircular canals has been described within the literature from various causes (i.e., the superior, horizontal [lateral], or posterior semicircular canal).[1] However, superior semicircular canal dehiscence is most commonly encountered.[1] The remainder of this chapter focuses on the clinical presentation, evaluation, and treatment of symptomatic superior semicircular canal dehiscence.

Superior semicircular canal dehiscence syndrome, or simply superior semicircular canal dehiscence, is a recently described process in which the superior bony covering separating the membranous labyrinth of the superior semicircular canal is in contact with the overlying dura of the middle

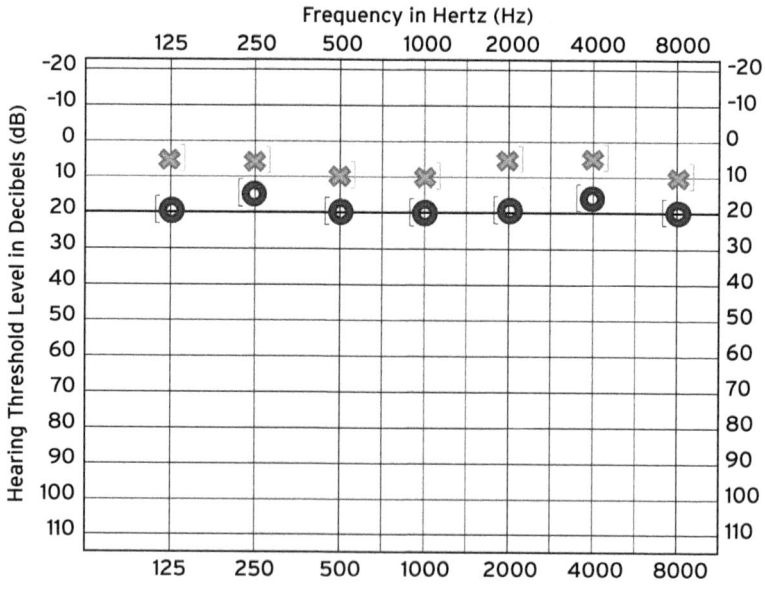

FIGURE 15-1 Pure tone audiogram from patient with pressure- and sound-induced vertigo. This patient presents with normal hearing on the left (x) and normal air conduction thresholds on the right (o). However, a right side small air bone gap is present.

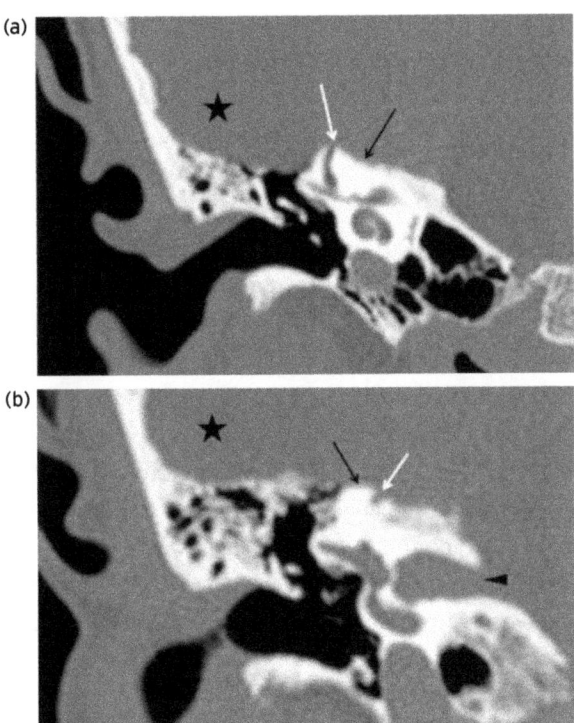

FIGURE 15-2 Coronal view CT of the temporal bones of the superior semicircular canal. The *black star* highlights the temporal lobe. The *white arrow* highlights the superior semicircular canal with apparent lack of bony covering. The *black arrow* depicts the dense bone of the otic capsule. The *arrowhead* depicts the internal auditory canal.

cranial fossa. Pressure changes in the middle fossa with change in intracranial pressure may be transmitted to the organs of the inner ear. The etiology of superior semicircular canal dehiscence is believed to be most commonly related to premature arrest in the development of the bone overlying the superior semicircular canal or congenital defects.[1] Interestingly, however, all patients with radiographic findings of superior semicircular canal dehiscence do not present symptomatically, nor do all individuals with postmortem confirmation findings of superior semicircular canal dehiscence have a past medical history consistent with symptomatic disease. The prevalence of superior semicircular canal dehiscence is approximately 0.5% based on cadaveric temporal bone analysis.[2,3] However, the exact prevalence of symptomatic superior semicircular canal dehiscence is unknown. No gender or racial predilection has been identified. Symptomatic semicircular canal dehiscence may present at any age.

CLINICAL PRESENTATION

The hallmark presentation of symptomatic superior semicircular canal dehiscence includes vertigo, oscillopsia, and hearing loss.[1] More specifically, patient may report vertigo or sensation of the world moving as if rotating on the face of a clock.[4] Patients may describe a sensation of vertical torsional motion.[4] The oscillopsia may be induced by loud sounds (Tullio phenomenon), changes in pressure in the ear canal transmitted to the middle ear (Hennebert sign), or with the Valsalva maneuver.[4-6] Normal environmental sounds have been noted to induce the oscillopsia, such as the dial tone on a telephone, a child's scream, or a church organ.[2,7] Dysequilibrium and motion intolerance in association with superior semicircular canal dehiscence has also been described.[4] Additionally, patients frequently present with auditory complaints. Patients may describe a sensation of hearing or feeling pulse in the affected ear, hearing eye movements, or hearing a heal strike the ground when running.[1,2,5,8] Autophony (hearing one's own voice) is commonly described.[1] Although vestibular complaints tend to predominate, patients may present primarily with auditory complaints.[9,10]

DIAGNOSTIC EVALUATION

In individuals presenting with superior semicircular canal dehiscence, the physical examination may reveal evoked eye movements with pneumatic otoscopy.[1] These eye movements are aligned with the canal of involvement (i.e., upward or torsional nystagmus with superior semicircular involvement). Additionally, the Valsalva maneuver may induce nystagmus by various mechanisms. A Valsalva maneuver against obstructed nostrils forces air into the middle ear through the eustachian tube resulting in inward displacement of the stapes. This produces excitatory motion of the semicircular canal ampulla. The Valsalva maneuver against a closed glottis (e.g., bearing down) causes increased intrathoracic pressure, decreased jugular venous return, and increased intracranial pressure leading to inhibitory motion of the superior semicircular canal.[11]

A tuning fork examination should be performed and may reveal "conductive hyperacusis." On examination, the Weber laterals to the affected ear.[1,2] Remarkably, patients may also hear a tuning fork placed on the lateral malleolus of the foot.[1,2]

Audiologic evaluation in this patient population may vary but typically identifies a conductive hearing loss (air-bone gap with normal bone conduction thresholds).[9] However, the presence of mild-to-moderate sensorineural hearing loss in association with superior semicircular canal dehiscence has been reported.[5] The speech discrimination scores, acoustic reflexes, and tympanometry are usually normal.[2,4,12] It is important to note that tympanometry may induce symptoms of vertigo.[6]

Electrophysiologic testing is commonly performed in patients with complaints of vertigo. Electronystagmography typically reveals no objective abnormal findings with loud sound or pressure because of the vertical or torsional nature of the nystagmus.[13] Similarly, caloric testing typically reveals normal findings.[8,14] In cases where a large dehiscence (i.e., >0.5 mm) is present, reduced vestibular function on the affected side has been reported.[3,15] It has been postulated that a large region of bony dehiscence allows the overlying dura of the temporal lobe to compress the membranous superior canal thereby impede the flow of endolymph leading to positive results on caloric testing.[6] Vestibular-evoked myogenic potentials, cervical or ocular, have been found to be useful in assessing patients with potential semicircular canal dehiscence.[2,8,9,16] A finding of decreased vestibular-evoked myogenic potentials threshold should increase the clinical suspicion regarding the diagnosis of superior semicircular canal dehiscence.[2,8,9,17]

A high-resolution coronal CT of the temporal bones with 1-mm cuts should be obtained in the plane of the vertical canal and usually identifies a dehiscence of the superior semicircular canal. Although the sensitivity of high-resolution CT of the temporal bone is quite high, this modality is associated with a low specificity and high false-positive rate for diagnosing superior semicircular canal dehiscence.[18] Most recently, 0.5-mm collimated multislice CT scan with reformation of images in the plane of the superior canal has been established, which possesses a higher specificity and positive predictive value in the diagnosis of superior semicircular canal dehiscence.[18]

Because of the constellation of symptoms associated with superior semicircular canal dehiscence, it has been deemed the great otologic mimicker. It has been reported that several patients with previously presumed perilymphatic fistula who underwent middle ear exploration and round window patching were truly suffering from symptoms in association with superior semicircular canal dehiscence.[4,5,13] Other otologic disease processes to be considered include patulous eustachian tube, Ménière's disease, and benign paroxysmal positional vertigo.[13,14,19]

TREATMENT

The treatment of semicircular canal dehiscence is predicated on the severity of symptoms. In individuals with mild symptoms, simple avoidance of triggering stimuli is sufficient. Alternatively, in patients with moderate symptoms, pressure equalization tube placement has been advocated to prevent increased middle ear pressure during Valsalva.[1] Operative repair is reserved for patients with debilitating disease.

Various approaches have been described for repair of superior semicircular canal dehiscence. The two main techniques for repair include resurfacing or plugging the superior semicircular canal.[4,5,8,14] Resurfacing of the superior semicircular canal may be achieved via a middle fossa craniotomy approach. In doing so, the abnormal connection between the membranous labyrinth and the middle fossa dura is alleviated. Various materials have been used for resurfacing including fibrin glue hydroxyapatite, fascia, conchal cartilage, bone, bone pate, and bone cement.[5] Additionally, via the middle fossa approach, superior semicircular canal plugging has been described in which fenestra are created in the superior semicircular canal on either side of the dehiscence followed by plugging with various material (e.g., bone pate or fascia).[4,5,8] Both techniques via the middle fossa approach have been found to be effective in alleviating or attenuating vestibular signs and symptoms.[4,5,8,12] In fact, complete resolution of symptoms is reported in most patients postoperatively at follow-up with marked decrease in symptoms reported by most of the remaining patients.[4,14] The most commonly reported persistent symptom within this patient population is dizziness with nose blowing.[11] Middle fossa approach repair has also demonstrated success in alleviating auditory symptoms.[9,20] The middle fossa approach repair is not without risk because it requires craniotomy and elevation of the temporal lobe to gain access to the superior semicircular canal. Additionally, a hospital stay with at least 1 day of intensive care services is required. This limits the patient population in which this approach is appropriate or desirable. Regardless of technique used, there is a significant risk of sensorineural hearing loss.[11]

Recently, less invasive alternative approaches have been described for repair or management of debilitating superior semicircular canal dehiscence symptoms, such as the transmastoid approach and round window occlusion. Via the transmastoid approach, superior semicircular canal resurfacing and plugging has been described.[21-24] Management of canal dehiscence via the transmastoid approach has been reported to have comparable results with those obtained via the middle fossa approach making the transmastoid approach quite favorable to patients and surgeons alike. The transmastoid approach alleviates the need for middle fossa craniotomy, does not require temporal bone retraction, and may be performed on an outpatient basis. However, in select groups of patients transmastoid approach is not feasible, most commonly secondary to low hanging dura of the middle fossa or extensive cranial base dehiscence requiring reconstruction.

Limited literature is available regarding the transcanal approach for management of semicircular canal dehiscence. The objective of this approach is not to repair or occlude the superior semicircular canal, but rather to alleviate the third window phenomenon postulated to contribute to the symptomatology of superior semicircular canal dehiscence. Within the transcanal approach, complete round window niche occlusion is employed using fascia, muscle, or fibrin glue.[25] This approach was born from the experience that patients later diagnosed with superior semicircular canal dehiscence that previously underwent middle ear exploration and round window occlusion without findings of perilymphatic fistula experienced alleviation of symptoms. Although there is anecdotal evidence supporting this approach, there remains a paucity of supportive evidence within the literature.

> **KEY POINTS TO REMEMBER**
> - The hallmark symptoms of superior semicircular canal dehiscence syndrome include vertigo, oscillopsia, and hearing loss
> - Tullio phenomenon may be present
> - Treatment is largely driven by the patient's tolerance of symptoms

Further Reading
1. Chien WW, Carey JP, Minor LB. Canal dehiscence. Curr Opin Neurol 2011;24:25–31.
2. Watson SR, Halmagyi GM, Colebatch JG. Vestibular hypersensitivity to sound. Tullio phenomenon: structural and functional assessment. Neurology 2000;54:722–8.
3. Carey JP, Minor LB, Nager GT. Dehiscence or thinning of bone overlying the superior semicircular canal in a temporal bone survey. Arch Otolaryngol Head Neck Surg 2000;126;137–47.
4. Minor LB, Solomon D, Zinreich JS, et al. Sound- and/or pressure-induced vertigo due to bone dehiscence of the superior semicircular canal. Arch Otolaryngol Head neck Surg 1998;124:246–58.
5. Minor LB. Superior canal dehiscence syndrome. Am J Otol 2000;21:9–19.
6. Minor LB, Cremer PD, Carey JP, et al. Symptoms and signs in superior semicircular canal dehiscence syndrome. Ann N Y Acad Sci 2001;942:259–73.
7. Ostrowski VB, Byskosh A, Hain TC. Tullio phenomenon with dehiscence of the superior semicircular canal. Otol Neurotol 2001;22:61–5.
8. Brantberg K, Bergenius J, Tribukait A. Vestibular-evoked myogenic potentials in patients with dehiscence of the superior semicircular canal. Acta Otolaryngol 1999;119:633–40.
9. Minor LB, Carey JP, Cremer PD, et al. Dehiscence of bone overlying the superior canal as a cause of apparent conductive hearing loss. Otol Neurotol 2003;24:270–8.
10. Mikulec AA, McKenna MJ, Ramsey MJ, et al. Superior semicircular canal dehiscence presenting as conductive hearing loss without vertigo. Otol Neurotol 2004;25:121–9.
11. Banerjee A, Whyte A, Atlas MD. Superior canal dehiscence: review of a new condition. Clin Otolaryngol 2005;30:9–15.
12. Brantberg K, Bergenius J, Mendel L, et al. Symptoms, findings, and treatment in patients with dehiscence of the superior semicircular canal. Acta Otolaryngol 2001;121:68–75.
13. Mong A, Loevner LA, Solomon D, et al. Sound- and pressure-induced vertigo associated with dehiscence of the roof of the superior semicircular canal. AJNR Am J Neuroradiol 1999;20:1973–5.
14. Smullen JL, Andrist EC, Gianoli GJ. Superior canal dehiscence: a new cause of vertigo. J La State Med Soc 1999;151:397–401.

15. Cremer PD, Minor LB, Carey JP, et al. Eye movements in patients with superior canal dehiscence syndrome align with abnormal canal. Neurology 2000;55:1833–41.
16. Welgampola MS, Myrie OA, Minor LB, Carey JP. Vestibular-evoked myogenic potential thresholds normalize on plugging superior canal dehiscence. Neurology 2008;70:464–72.
17. Aw ST, Todd MJ, Aw GE, et al. Click-evoked vestibulo-ocular reflex: stimulus-response properties in superior canal dehiscence. Neurology 2006;66:1079–87.
18. Belden CJ, Weg N, Minor LB, et al. CT evaluation of bone dehiscence of the superior semicircular canal as a cause of sound- and/or pressure-induced vertigo. Radiology 2003;226:337–43.
19. Zhou G, Gopen Q, Poe DS. Clinical and diagnostic characterization of canal dehiscence syndrome: a great otologic mimicker. Otol Neurotol 2007;28:920–6.
20. Crane BT, Lin FR, Minor LB, Carey JP. Improvement in autophony symptoms after superior canal dehiscence repair. Otol Neurotol 2010;31:140–6.
21. Agrawal SK, Parnes LS. Transmastoid superior semicircular canal occlusion. Otol Neurotol 2008;29:363–7.
22. Crovetto M, Areitio E, Elexpuru J, Aguayo F. Transmastoid approach for resurfacing of superior semicircular canal dehiscence. Auris Nasus Larynx 2008;35:247–9.
23. Deschenes GR, Hsu DP, Megerian CA. Outpatient repair of superior semicircular canal dehiscence via the transmastoid approach. Laryngoscope 2009;119:1765–9.
24. Kirtane MV, Sharma A, Satwalekar D. Transmastoid repair of superior semicircular canal dehiscence. J Laryngol Otol 2009;123:356–8.
25. Silverstein H, Van Ess MJ. Complete round window niche occlusion for superior semicircular canal dehiscence syndrome: a minimally invasive approach. Ear Nose Throat J 2009;88:1042–56.

16 Labyrinthine Concussion

A 36-year-old male presents for evaluation of vertigo and instability. Symptoms began approximately 2 days following a motor vehicle accident in which he sustained head trauma. He was an unrestrained passenger and struck his head on the dashboard. He suffered brief loss of consciousness, but does remember being transported to the hospital. He sustained lacerations to his forehead that were repaired in the emergency department.
A computed tomography (CT) of the head was obtained revealing no evidence of injury to the cranial vault, facial fractures, or intracranial hemorrhage. Onset of constant vertigo occurred approximately 3 days following the accident and he was treated with antiemetics and vestibular suppressants. He presents 3 weeks following the accident for evaluation of residual symptoms of vertigo and instability. The vertigo now has a positional association. He notes difficulty with stability particularly navigating to the bathroom in the middle of the night. He denies hearing loss, neck pain, headache, photophobia, phonophobia, or vision changes. The past medical history is significant for asthma for which he takes albuterol as needed. Physical examination reveals right gaze nystagmus, a positive Romberg sign, and difficulty with tandem gait. On tuning fork examination, the Weber is midline and the Rinne is positive (air conduction greater than bone). Review of images from CT of head confirms lack of intracranial pathology or fractures. An audiogram revealed normal hearing at the low frequencies with a mild sensorineural hearing loss at the high frequencies on the right. Speech discrimination scores were 100% bilaterally. Electronystagmography (ENG) revealed a 35% decreased vestibular response on the right. Magnetic resonance imaging of the internal auditory canal and posterior skull base revealed normal findings with the exception of high signal from the otic labyrinth on preconstrast imaging.

What do you do now?

Vertigo following head trauma is exceedingly common. The incidence of vertigo posttrauma has been reported to range from 15% to 78% depending on criteria used.[1-5] Most cases involving vertigo post head trauma are associated with motor vehicle accidents followed by assaults and falls.[6]

Various etiologies have been identified in association with posttraumatic vertigo including brainstem concussion, eighth nerve complex injury, posttraumatic Ménière's disease, delayed endolymphatic hydrops, rupture of round window, perilymphatic fistula, labyrinthine concussion, otic capsule violating temporal bone fracture, benign paroxysmal positional vertigo, postconcussion syndrome, whiplash injury syndrome, epileptic vertigo, diffuse axonal injury, posttraumatic migraine, and psychogenic vertigo. Labyrinthine concussion is one of the most common etiologies for posttraumatic vertigo.

Labyrinthine concussion was first described over a century ago.[7-10] The diagnosis of labyrinthine concussion precludes the presence of ipsilateral temporal bone fracture with otic capsule violation. Vertigo in those instances is attributable to disruption of the bony labyrinthine capsule. However, labyrinthine concussion most commonly occurs ipsilateral to an otic capsule sparing temporal bone fractures (i.e., bony labyrinthine capsule remains intact and uninvolved in the fracture), but it may occur contralateral to temporal bone trauma or in patients without temporal bone fracture.[9-11]

Labyrinthine concussion is typically associated with parietal-occipital or temporal-parietal vector of trauma force.[12] However, the pathophysiology of labyrinthine concussion is not well understood. Various proposed pathophysiologic mechanisms have been described including the following:

1. A posthemorrhagic inflammatory response leading to the deposition of fibrous tissue and osteoneogenesis[13]
2. Traumatic vasomotor changes in the inner ear affecting microcirculation of the vestibular organ[7,14]
3. Disruption of inner ear microcirculation secondary to small clots affecting the vestibular organ[15]
4. Physical disruption of the sensory epithelium by traumatic pressure waves transmitted from the intracranial cerebrospinal fluid to the inner ear[10,16]

5. Local hypoxia leading to biochemical alteration in the fluid of the inner ear causing damage to sensory epithelium[14,17]

There is no gender or racial predilection for the development of labyrinthine concussion following head trauma. Although most studies describing labyrinthine concussion focus on the adult population, labyrinthine concussion has been documented to also occur within the pediatric population.[12]

CLINICAL PRESENTATION

Labyrinthine concussion presents following head trauma, but the degree of preceding trauma may range from mild to severe. Loss of consciousness during the episode of trauma is often reported.[10] The symptoms may present immediately, but most commonly present several days following the injury. During the acute phase, patients present with vertigo of varied severity with associated nausea and emesis. During the subacute or chronic phases a sense of imbalance and constant instability may be reported. Symptoms tend to worsen with fatigue or in dark environments. Additionally, positional vertigo in the subacute or chronic phase may be encountered.

Patients with labyrinthine concussion may present with varied auditory status ranging from normal hearing to profound sensorineural hearing loss. However, typically patients present with normal hearing or only mild hearing loss. Complaints of more severe hearing loss should increase the clinical suspicion of occult temporal bone fracture with otic capsule involvement, ossicular discontinuity, or disturbance of the proximal auditory pathway prompting further diagnostic evaluation including imaging of the temporal bone and skull base.

DIAGNOSTIC EVALUATION

On physical examination, patients with labyrinthine concussion in the acute phase may present with diaphoresis, pallor, nausea, and emesis. Gaze nystagmus is often present. Tuning fork examination should be performed to assess for asymmetric hearing and sensorineural versus conductive hearing loss. These patients may present with a positive Romberg sign and gait ataxia. During the later phases, gaze nystagmus often resolves. However, nystagmus may be inducible with positional association. The Dix-Hallpike may be positive in these patients making it challenging to differentiate benign paroxysmal positional vertigo from labyrinthine concussion or combined disease in the chronic phase. Vertigo and nystagmus induced by Valsalva maneuver, pneumatic otoscopy (Hennebert's sign), or loud sounds (Tullio phenomenon) should raise the clinical suspicion for alternative diagnoses. It is important to note that labyrinthine concussion is commonly associated with or is followed by additional vestibulopathies including benign paroxysmal positional vertigo, central vestibular disorder, and cervicogenic vertigo.[18] The presence of signs or symptoms supporting an alternative diagnosis does not entirely preclude labyrinthine concussion as being a contributing factor to the patient's presentation.

With complaints of hearing loss or abnormalities noted on tuning fork examination, formal audiometric evaluation should be performed including pure tone audiometry and speech discrimination. Patients with labyrinthine concussion typically present with normal hearing or mild-to-moderate high-frequency sensorineural hearing loss. However, because of the high rate of association with additional injuries, conductive hearing loss or more severe sensorineural hearing loss may be observed.

Vestibular assessment should be performed in these patients including ENG or videonystagmography (VNG). Hypofunction is commonly associated with the presentation of labyrinthine concussion.[19] Among patients with vertigo and postural instability, in a study by Nacci and coworkers[20] in 2011, 11% of patients postwhiplash injury and 50% of patients following minor head trauma exhibited vestibular hypofunction on caloric evaluation. Overall within the literature, abnormal caloric response and hypofunction on ENG/VNG following head injury range from 32% to 71%.[2-5,21-24] Complete absence of vestibular response on ENG/VNG is not characteristic of labyrinthine concussion. Rotational chair assessment may be performed if there is ambiguity regarding the diagnosis or to assist in clinical decision making regarding treatment. On rotational chair assessment pathologic results for a peripheral lesion are noted.[18] Vestibulospinal testing reveals deviation to the side of injury.[18]

Imaging of the head and temporal bone are an important component of the diagnostic evaluation of patients with vertigo following head trauma. CT of the temporal bones should be obtained to evaluate for temporal bone fracture or intracranial hemorrhage. Magnetic resonance imaging is less commonly used as a first-line imaging modality. However, it has been demonstrated to be of benefit in demonstrating labyrinthine hemorrhage.[25]

NATURAL HISTORY

Symptoms in association with labyrinthine concussion may have an early onset following trauma, but typically present several days later. The initial phase of disease is one of vertigo, nausea, and emesis. This typically resolves within days to weeks following the injury and is replaced by a sensation of instability. Occasional episodes of vertigo or positionally associated vertigo may present in the chronic phase of disease. In most cases, with central compensation, these symptoms abate and are self-limited. However, in patients with concomitant central injury, dysfunction of additional vestibular mechanisms (i.e., vision and proprioception), and advanced age these symptoms may remain long-term.

TREATMENT

Labyrinthine concussion in most cases represents a self-limited disease. As such, in most patients treatment is largely supportive. Within the acute phase, vestibular suppressants and antiemetics may be prescribed for symptomatic relief. Caution and care should be taken regarding the duration of vestibular suppressant use because it may retard central compensation of vestibular hypofunction. With most patients, supportive care followed by vestibular physical therapy is successful in assisting patients to return to their baseline level of function.

In a select group of patients, chronic symptoms of instability or episodic vertigo remain present in association with labyrinthine concussion. In these patients surgical intervention may be an option. Denervation on the involved side has been described in the literature, namely labyrinthectomy (chemical or surgical), in patients with nonserviceable hearing. Vestibular nerve section may be performed in individuals with serviceable hearing.[26,27] A complete vestibular assessment, including rotational chair assessment, must be performed prior to denervation to ensure the integrity of the visual and proprioceptive systems, which are required for central compensation. In patients posttrauma, these systems may also be deficient. Additionally, central dysfunction is common following head trauma with up to 60% having central vestibular deficit.[5] This presence of central, visual, or proprioceptive dysfunction may significantly hinder central compensation. Additionally, advanced age can impact central vestibular compensation; thus, denervation within the elderly should be performed with extreme caution. The final consideration regarding denervation pertains to symptoms experienced by the patient. Even in the presence of reduced vestibular response on ENG or VNG, denervation should only be embarked on in patients with active symptoms of vertigo. A poor prognosis for resolution of symptoms has been reported following denervation in patients with vestibular hypofunction and instability without vertigo.[27]

KEY POINTS TO REMEMBER

- Vertigo following head trauma is common
- Labyrinthine concussion is typically associated with parietal-occipital or temporal-parietal trauma
- Labyrinthine concussion in most cases is self-limited

Further Reading

1. Berman JM, Frederickson JM. Vertigo after head injury: a five-year follow up. J Otolaryngol 1978;7:237–45.
2. Toglia JU, Rosenberg PE, Ronis ML. Posttraumatic dizziness; vestibular, audiologic and medico-legal aspects. Arch Otolaryngol 1970;92:485–92.
3. Barber HO. Head injury-audiological and vestibular findings. Ann Otol Rhinol Laryngol 1969;78:239–52.
4. Rutherford WH. Sequelae of concussion caused by minor head injuries. Lancet 1977;1:1–4.
5. Tuohimaa P. Vestibular disturbances after acute mild head injury. Acta Otolaryngol Suppl 1978;359:3–67.
6. Bernstein DM. Recovering from mild head injury. Brain Inj 1999;13:151–72.
7. Brunner H. Commotio auris internae. In: Alexander HV, Marburg O, editors: Handbuch Neurologie des Ohres. Munich: Urban & Schwarzenberg, 1928. p 37.

8. Voss O. Is there a labyrinthine concussion? JAMA 1934;103:1721–2.
9. Schuknecht HF, Davison RC. Deafness and vertigo from head injury. AMA Arch Otolaryngol 1956;63:513–28.
10. Schuknecht HF. Mechanisms of inner ear injury from blows to the head. Ann Otol Rhinol Laryngol 1969;78:253–62.
11. Davey LM. Labyrinthine trauma in head injury. Conn Med 1965;29:250–3.
12. Eviatar L, Bergtraum M, Randel RM. Post-traumatic vertigo in children: a diagnostic approach. Pediatr Neurol 1986;2:61–6.
13. Lindsay JR, Zajtchuk J. Concussion of the inner ear. Ann Otol Rhinol Laryngol 1970;79:699–709.
14. Fitzgerald DC. Head trauma: hearing loss and dizziness. J Trauma 1996;40:488–96.
15. Axelsson A, Hallen C. The healing of the external cochlear wall in guinea pig after mechanical trauma. Arch Otolaryngol 1973;76:136–48.
16. Makishima K, Snow JB Jr. Electrophysiological responses from the cochlea and inferior colliculus in guinea pigs after head trauma. Laryngoscope 1975;85:1947–57.
17. Ilberg CV. Inner ear hearing loss following blunt head injury [author's transl]. Laryngol Rhinol Otol (Stuttg) 1977;56:323–8.
18. Ernst A, Basta D, Seidl RO, et al. Management of posttraumatic vertigo. Otolaryngol Head Neck Surg 2005;132:554–8.
19. Lachman J. The importance of vestibular examination in post-concussion vertigo. Acta Med Orient 1955;14:44–66.
20. Nacci A, Ferrazzi M, Berrettini S, et al. Vestibular and stabilometric findings in whiplash injury and minor head trauma. Acta Otorhinolaryngol Ital 2011;31:378–89.
21. Compere WE Jr. Electronystagmographic findings in patients with "whiplash injuries." Laryngoscope 1968;78:1226–33.
22. Rubin W. Whiplash with vestibular involvement. Arch Otolaryngol 1975;97:85–7.
23. Oosterveld WJ, Kortschot HW, Kingma GG, et al. Electronystagmographic findings following cervical whiplash injuries. Acta Otolaryngol 1991;111:201–5.
24. Akin FW, Murnane OD. Head injury and blast exposure: vestibular consequences. Otolaryngol Clin N Am 2011;44:323–34.
25. Weissman JL, Curtin HD, Hirsch BE, et al. High signal from the otic labyrinth on unenhanced magnetic resonance imaging. AJNR AM J Neuroradiol 1992;13:1183–7.
26. Kemink JL, Telian SA, Graham MD, et al. Transmastoid labyrinthectomy: reliable surgical management of vertigo. Otolaryngol Head Neck Surg 1989;101:5–10.
27. Sanna M, Ylikosky J. Vestibular neurectomy for dizziness after head trauma. A review of 28 patients. ORL J Otorhinolaryngol Relat Spec 1983;45:216–25.

SECTION III

Tinnitus

17 Subjective Tinnitus

A 57-year-old male presents with disturbing high-pitched tinnitus that interferes with sleep and concentration. The tinnitus is perceived in both ears, but louder in the left ear. It has been present for a few months. It is louder in quiet and with clenching his teeth. He played drums in a rock band from his early 20s to his 40s, but denies hearing loss (HL). Past medical history is significant for hyperlipidemia. There is no past surgical or trauma history. Medications include a statin drug, a baby aspirin, and once-weekly use of a phosphodiesterase (PDE-5) inhibitor for erectile dysfunction. He does not use tobacco, he drinks one to two gin-and-tonics three to four times per week, he does not use recreational drugs, he drinks two large cups of coffee and two caffeinated sodas daily, he eats a diet of 3,500 mg of sodium daily, and he drinks one glass of water per day. Physical examination is significant only for mild discomfort with deep palpation of the temporomandibular joints (TMJs) bilaterally.

What do you do now?

Subjective tinnitus affects 30 million people in the United States, and is considered disabling or nearly disabling by one-quarter of those.[1] Degree of tinnitus-related quality of life (QOL) impairment varies greatly. Assessing QOL related to tinnitus at initial evaluation, and using that same measure at the conclusion of therapy, is very helpful for assessing utility of treatment and treatment response, and to help the patient see their own progress. The Tinnitus Handicap Inventory (Table 17-1) is a self-reported measure answering 25 questions as "yes," "sometimes," or "no."[2] "Yes" is scored as 4 points; "sometimes" as 2 points, and "no" as 0 points. The higher the score on the Tinnitus Handicap Inventory, the more handicapped the patient is from their tinnitus. If patients are minimally or mildly affected by their tinnitus, explanation of possible causes and possible exacerbators, with minor dietary or other modifications, is usually sufficient. If the Tinnitus Handicap Inventory reveals a large number of psychiatric issues, consultation with the appropriate mental health provider is important. Overall, the Tinnitus Handicap Inventory is valid for both initial and later assessment, and for communication with the patient.

Subjective tinnitus, or head noise or phantom head noise, can be perceived in varying ways. Although it is frequently described as a ringing or a high-pitched whine, it may also resemble a hiss, a radiator sound, a seashore sound, a clanging, or a low roar. Musical tinnitus may be a clearly central nervous system–mediated phenomenon. An international methodologic standard for tinnitus trials has been proposed.[3] For the clinician, it is important to have an accurate representation of the tinnitus perception and its intensity and affect on QOL.

Tinnitus may result from several causes. It is primarily important to rule out HL, even if the patient is not aware, because tinnitus is often perceived in the presence of HL. Both presbycusis and noise-induced HL (NIHL) usually affect high-frequency hearing. The patient may not notice the HL at all, or may note difficulty in *understanding* but not difficulty in *hearing*, because high-frequency sensorineural HL affects perception of consonants. Hearing screen with a 512-Hz tuning fork is, therefore, not adequate. A formal audiogram (that includes determination of word recognition score) should be performed. Figure 17-1 shows a typical audiogram of a patient with NIHL. Otoacoustic emissions testing may also be helpful.

TABLE 17-1 **Tinnitus Handicap Inventory**

1 Because of your tinnitus is it difficult to concentrate?	Yes	Sometimes	No
2 Does the loudness of your tinnitus make it difficult for you to hear people?	Yes	Sometimes	No
3 Does your tinnitus make you angry?	Yes	Sometimes	No
4 Does your tinnitus make you feel confused?	Yes	Sometimes	No
5 Because of your tinnitus do you feel desperate?	Yes	Sometimes	No
6 Do you complain a great deal about your tinnitus?	Yes	Sometimes	No
7 Because of your tinnitus do you have trouble falling asleep at night?	Yes	Sometimes	No
8 Do you feel that you cannot escape your tinnitus?	Yes	Sometimes	No
9 Does your tinnitus interfere with your ability to enjoy social activities (such as going out to dinner, to the movies)?	Yes	Sometimes	No
10 Because of your tinnitus do you feel frustrated?	Yes	Sometimes	No
11 Because of your tinnitus do you feel that you have a terrible disease?	Yes	Sometimes	No
12 Does your tinnitus make it difficult for you to enjoy life?	Yes	Sometimes	No
13 Does your tinnitus interfere with your job or household duties?	Yes	Sometimes	No
14 Because of your tinnitus do you find that you are often irritable?	Yes	Sometimes	No
15 Because of your tinnitus is it difficult for you to read?	Yes	Sometimes	No
16 Does your tinnitus make you upset?	Yes	Sometimes	No
17 Do you feel that your tinnitus problem has placed stress on your relationship with members of your family and friends?	Yes	Sometimes	No
18 Do you find it difficult to focus your attention away from your tinnitus and on other things?	Yes	Sometimes	No

(continued)

TABLE 17-1 **(Continued)**

19	Do you feel that you have no control over your tinnitus?	Yes	Sometimes	No
20	Because of your tinnitus do you often feel tired?	Yes	Sometimes	No
21	Because of your tinnitus do you feel depressed?	Yes	Sometimes	No
22	Does your tinnitus make you feel anxious?	Yes	Sometimes	No
23	Do you feel that you can no longer cope with your tinnitus?	Yes	Sometimes	No
24	Does your tinnitus get worse when you are under stress?	Yes	Sometimes	No
25	Does your tinnitus make you feel insecure?	Yes	Sometimes	No

Yes = 4; Sometimes = 2; No = 0.

Asymmetric otologic symptoms or findings always merit consideration of retrocochlear pathology. This is even if the patient states that their only source of NIHL came from the worse-hearing side. If the hearing level at 4 kHz is better than (less than) 80 dB, an auditory brainstem response test, also known as brainstem evoked response audiometry, can be performed. Auditory brainstem response is accurate in diagnosing nearly 100% of acoustic neuromas (vestibular schwannomas) sized 2 cm or larger, but may miss up to 19% of intracanalicular tumors less than 1 cm in size.[4] A gadolinium-enhanced magnetic resonance imaging (MRI) study through the brain and internal auditory canals is currently considered the gold standard for retrocochlear diagnosis, and may also show other pathologies, such as multiple sclerosis or siderosis, which may present as tinnitus. A less expensive MRI modality that avoids the use of gadolinium is a T2 fast spin echo study, which has equal sensitivity for internal auditory canal pathology but may miss other brain pathologies.[5] If the patient cannot have MRI, computed tomography scan of the brain and internal auditory canals with and without contrast is recommended. If the patient opts not to have either auditory brainstem response or computed tomography or MRI, he or she should have a follow-up audiogram in 6 months at the very least, and such conversation should be documented in the chart.[6] Other types of brain imaging (positron emission tomography or functional MRI) are used in research and not yet clinically applicable.

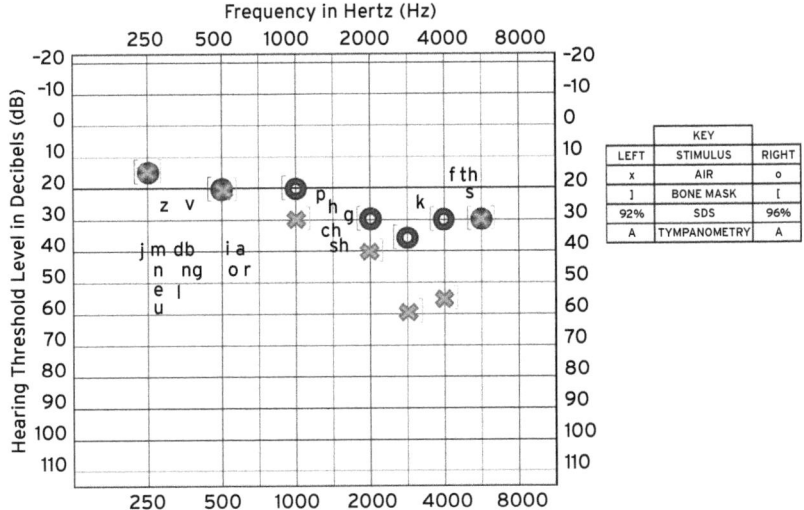

FIGURE 17-1 Audiogram of patient with asymmetric noise-induced hearing loss (HL). Typical noise-induced pattern of high-frequency sensorineural HL with worse hearing (dip) at 3–4 kHz to a severe sensorineural HL level with "recovery" to mild sensorineural HL at the higher frequencies in the left ear, and a dip only to mild sensorineural HL in the right ear. Although word recognition score is excellent bilaterally, that is tested in quiet. This patient likely has difficulty understanding terminal consonant sounds ("f," "s," "k," and "th"), particularly in background noise. He would likely "match" his tinnitus to around 4000 Hz.

For imaging considerations, subjective tinnitus should be divided into pulsatile and nonpulsatile. Imaging of nonpulsatile tinnitus is indicated for asymmetry, as discussed previously. Pulsatile tinnitus suggests a vascular neoplasm, vascular anomaly, or vascular malformation. Dural vascular malformations are often elusive on all cross-sectional imaging studies; conventional angiography may be necessary. Flow-sensitive MRI can show vascular loops compressing the eighth cranial nerve. Carotid dissections, aneurysms, atherosclerosis, and fibromuscular dysplasia can be identified on MRI or MR angiographic studies and computed tomography or computed tomography angiographic studies.[7] Pulsatile tinnitus, although much more uncommon that nonpulsatile tinnitus, is discussed in detail in subsequent chapters.

TMJ arthalgia or cervical myalgia may cause or exacerbate subjective tinnitus. Treatment of the underlying musculoskeletal dysfunction can be curative or at least very helpful in management of tinnitus.[8]

Statin drugs do not typically cause ototoxicity. There is only one case report of tinnitus and HL from a statin.[9] Low-dose aspirin is also not ototoxic. However, PDE-5 inhibitors may be associated with HL of which tinnitus is a corresponding symptom.[10] Temporal relation of otologic symptoms to ingestion of the PDE-5 inhibitor is helpful but not necessary.

This patient's social history raises a number of red flags. Caffeine and nicotine, as vasoconstrictors, are frequent culprits in heightening the experience of tinnitus. Reduction or elimination of, in this case, caffeine consumption would likely afford significant tinnitus relief or even complete resolution. An "otologically healthy" diet contains less than 2,500 mg of sodium per day; however, there are no data supporting low-salt diet in treatment of tinnitus. Inadequate hydration is also considered otologically unsound and is generally considered, with a small amount of literature to support it,[11] a potential cause of tinnitus. Tonic water contains up to 83 ppm (milligrams per liter) of quinine. In a study, even a single dose of 300 mg of quinine caused (reversible) HL in 75% of otherwise healthy individuals.[12] Heavy, regular consumption, such as is reported by this patient, should alert the physician and elimination of quinine should be part of the initial treatment protocol.

Insomnia or other poor sleep patterns exacerbate tinnitus. Anxiety, depression, and somatiform disorders are associated with tinnitus. Medical treatment of the underlying psychiatrist illness, and directed to the insomnia, along with cognitive behavioral therapy, can be very beneficial in these patients.[13]

Treatment considerations for the patient with subjective tinnitus should be organized methodically into (1) understanding of situation, (2) elimination of ototoxins, (3) medical and cognitive behavioral treatment, (4) use of devices, and (5) more invasive treatments.

1. *Understanding.* The patient with subjective tinnitus is often scared or confused, and may have received inadequate information from prior physicians. Explaining the relationship between his or her sensorineural HL and tinnitus is very helpful, including the statement that tinnitus is a brain phenomenon that is believed to be a central nervous system reinterpretation of "remembered" cochlear microphonics. Explaining the relationship between

stress/anxiety/insomnia, and caffeine/nicotine/dehydration/ other toxins, and increased tinnitus is also helpful. An analogy that is very conducive to improved understanding and shared decision-making is the following. "The goal is to make your tinnitus be like your socks and shoes. Your brain does not waste all day informing you that you are wearing socks and shoes. That is our goal at the conclusion of these treatments: that you may still have tinnitus, but you don't waste any more time or energy paying attention to it."

2. *Elimination of Ototoxins.* First-line treatment is minimizing or eliminating caffeine, nicotine, dehydration, and any potentially ototoxic substances.

3. *Medical and Cognitive Behavioral Treatment.* Several medications and herbal agents have been used, with varying degrees of success. These include low-dose clonazepam (0.25–0.5 mg at bedtime), gabapentin, anxiolytics, antidepressants, *Gingko biloba*, and melatonin. *N*-Acetylcysteine is shown to reduce acute-onset NIHL and potentially the secondary tinnitus.[14] Treatments should also be geared to underlying anxiety or depression. Cognitive behavioral therapy, known as tinnitus-retraining therapy, is a labor-intensive modality. In extensive reviews, antidepressants and tinnitus-retraining therapy are the only of these treatments with adequate evidence in the literature.[15,16] Sleep disturbances should be identified and treated aggressively. Treatment of TMJ and cervical arthralgia, when identified, is appropriate.

4. *Use of Devices.* When HL is identified, appropriate fitting of hearing aids alone or with ear-level masking devices should be considered, because hearing aids themselves "resolve" the perceived tinnitus in more than 50% of patients.[17] If HL is not present, ear-level maskers alone may be used, or "white," "pink," or other types of masking noises may be introduced into the environment. Other devices that are approved for tinnitus include the Neuromonics™ tinnitus treatment device, phase-shifting devices, and transcranial magnetic stimulation. None of these have overwhelming evidence for success; however,

when targeted to properly selected patients, they may be of benefit.

5. *More Invasive Treatments.* Intratympanic injection of steroids, aminoglycosides, or lidocaine for tinnitus relief is successful in some percentage of patients. Side effect profiles and resultant HL are considerations.[18] Cochlear implantation for tinnitus relief is being investigated. Cochlear nerve section has been performed in the past to alleviate disabling tinnitus; this is not an effective treatment.

Contrary to widely held beliefs, a targeted treatment program can be beneficial in up to 85%–90% of patients.[19] It is important that the patient's complaint of tinnitus be addressed, because relatively simple maneuvers can be of great benefit. If the tinnitus becomes disabling, a multifaceted approach to care that includes otologic care, avoidance of toxins, device use, medications for sleep, anxiety, depression, psychiatric or psychological care, habituation, and even more invasive maneuvers, can significantly improve QOL in these patients.

KEY POINTS TO REMEMBER

- Audiometric evaluation can aid in assessment of patients with subjective tinnitus.
- Use of validated questionnaires, such as the Dizziness Handicap Index, helps distinguish between disabling, bothersome, and nonbothersome tinnitus.
- Imaging studies are indicated to rule out retrocochlear pathology in nonpulsatile tinnitus with asymmetric HL.
- Musculoskeletal dysfunction, such as TMJ arthralgia or cervical myalgia, may cause or exacerbate tinnitus.
- Treatments include restriction of caffeine and nicotine intake; avoidance of potentially ototoxic substances, such as high-dose aspirin and quinine; and several other treatments, including treatment of insomnia and psychiatric intervention if appropriate

Further Reading

1. Kochkin S, Tyler R, Born J. MarkeTrak VIII: the prevalence of tinnitus in the United States and the self-reported efficacy of various treatments. Hear Rev 2011;18(12):10–27. See more at: http://www.hearingreview.com/2011/11/marketrak-viii-the-prevalence-of-tinnitus-in-the-united-states-and-the-self-reported-efficacy-of-various-treatments/#sthash.YieP84Wn.dpuf
2. McCombe A, Bagueley D, Coles R, McKenna L, McKinney C, Windle-Taylor P. Guidelines for the grading of tinnitus severity: the results of a working group commissioned by the British Association of Otolaryngologists, Head and Neck Surgeons, 1999. Clin Otolaryngol 2001;26:388–93.
3. Landgrebe M, Azevedo A, Baguley D, et al. Methodological aspects of clinical trials in tinnitus: a proposal for an international standard. J Psychosom Res 2012;73:112–21.
4. Chandrasekhar SS, Brackmann DE, Devgan KK. Utility of auditory brainstem response audiometry in diagnosis of acoustic neuromas. Am J Otol 1995;16:63–7.
5. Daniels RL, Swallow C, Shelton C, Davidson HC, Krejci CS, Harnsberger HR. Causes of unilateral sensorineural hearing loss screened by high-resolution fast spin echo magnetic resonance imaging: review of 1,070 consecutive cases. Am J Otol 2000;21:173–80.
6. Stachler RJ, Chandrasekhar SS, Archer SM, et al. Clinical practice guideline: sudden hearing loss. Otolaryngol Head Neck Surg 2012;146(suppl 3):S1–35.
7. Weissman JL, Hirsch BE. Imaging of tinnitus: a review. Radiology 2000;216:342.
8. Björne A. Assessment of temporomandibular and cervical spine disorders in tinnitus patients. Prog Brain Res 2007;166:215–9.
9. Liu M, Alafris A, Longo AJ, Cohen H. Irreversible atorvastatin-associated hearing loss. Pharmacotherapy 2012;32:e27–34.
10. Maddox PT, Saunders J, Chandrasekhar SS. Sudden hearing loss from PDE-5 inhibitors: a possible cellular stress etiology. Laryngoscope 2009;119:1586–9.
11. Sakata E, Sakata H. Special features of old age vertigo. Int Tinnitus J 2001;7:115–7.
12. Claessen FA, van Boxtel CJ, Perenboom RM, Tange RA, Wetsteijn JC, Kager PA. Quinine pharmacokinetics: ototoxic and cardiotoxic effects in healthy Caucasian subjects and in patients with falciparum malaria. Trop Med Int Health 1998;3:482–9.
13. Belli H, Belli S, Oktay MF, Ural C. Psychopathological dimensions of tinnitus and psychopharmacologic approaches in its treatment. Gen Hosp Psychiatry 2012;34:282–9.
14. Kopke RD, Jackson RL, Coleman JK, Liu J, Bielefeld EC, Balough BJ. NAC for noise: from the bench top to the clinic. Hear Res 2007;226):114–25.
15. Hoare DJ, Kowalkowski VL, Kang S, Hall DA. Systematic review and meta-analyses of randomized controlled trials examining tinnitus management. Laryngoscope 2011;121:1555–64.
16. Bauer CA, Brozoski TJ. Effect of tinnitus retraining therapy on the loudness and annoyance of tinnitus: a controlled trial. Ear Hear 2011;32:145–55.

17. Hobson J, Chisholm E, El Refaie A. Sound therapy (masking) in the management of tinnitus in adults. Cochrane Database Syst Rev 2010;8:CD006371.
18. Dodson KM, Sismanis A. Intratympanic perfusion for the treatment of tinnitus. Otolaryngol Clin North Am 2004;37:991–1000.
19. Shulman A, Goldstein B. Principles of tinnitology: tinnitus diagnosis and treatment a tinnitus-targeted therapy. Int Tinnitus J 2010;16:73–85.

18 Paragangliomas

A 37-year-old female presents with a several month history of pulsatile right-sided tinnitus with hearing loss. She has also noted progressive breathiness and hoarseness, with inability to project her voice. This is affecting her profession as an elementary school teacher. She occasionally chokes when she drinks liquids, and she sometimes has difficulty pronouncing words with the tip of her tongue. Past history and family history are all negative. Social history is significant for one to two glasses of red wine per week, one cup of coffee per day, no tobacco use, normal salt diet, four to five glasses of water per day, and no use of illegal drugs. Physical examination reveals a thin female with a breathy voice and no dyspnea. There is a pulsating reddish mass seen in the posterior-inferior aspect of the right middle ear, behind the tympanic membrane. The mass blanches with positive air pressure (or insufflation). The protruded tongue deviates to the right. Right shoulder shrug is weak. Laryngoscopy reveals right true vocal fold paralysis. Tuning forks demonstrate conductive hearing loss on the right. The remaining cranial nerves (CNs) are normal. There are no bruits or thrills in the neck.

What do you do now?

Jugulotympanic paragangliomas (also known as glomus tumors) are benign neuroendocrine tumors. Glomus tympanicum (GT) and glomus jugulare (GJ) are paragangliomas that present in the temporal bone. These tumors may present with pulsatile tinnitus, conductive hearing loss, and CN neuropathy.

Accurate diagnosis is the first step in managing these patients. Physical examination reveals the diagnosis in most cases. The most common physical sign in paraganglioma diagnosis is a vascular middle ear mass. The differential diagnosis is somewhat limited. A high-riding jugular bulb is usually posterior and blue in color, and is not pulsatile. A facial nerve neuroma is usually along the lie of the fallopian canal and is generally less vascular. Aberrant internal carotid artery is more anterior in the mesotympanum. Primary neoplasms of the middle ear, such as an adenoma, are not pulsatile. Pneumatic otoscopy results in a Brown's sign in 10%–30% of glomus tumors, which is blanching of the paraganglioma on air insufflation with secondary temporary compression of the tumor. Audiometric evaluation shows either conductive or mixed hearing loss, and tympanogram may be able to capture the pulsations of the tumor.

Imaging begins with noncontrast high-resolution computed tomography (CT) of the temporal bone, performed in the axial and coronal planes. In most cases, CT confirms the distinction between GT and GJ (Figure 18-1). Magnetic resonance imaging with and without gadolinium enhancement is effective for delineating extent of GJ tumor in the mastoid and in the neck and its relationship with the dura (Figure 18-2). Angiography is generally combined with embolization as a preoperative modality (Figure 18-3).

GT tumors are limited to the middle ear space and mastoid. Their origin is usually on the medial wall of the middle ear, from glomus bodies accompanying the tympanic (Jacobson's) nerve through the middle ear.[1]

When diagnosed early, they can often be "shelled" out via transcanal middle ear surgery with no sequelae. Larger tumors require mastoidectomy and possibly extended facial recess approach.[2] Surgical removal is the recommended treatment modality.

GJ tumors arise from glomus bodies in the wall of the jugular nerve. They are often very large by the time of presentation, often referred to as a "rising sun" appearance on otoscopy. Because they arise in the jugular

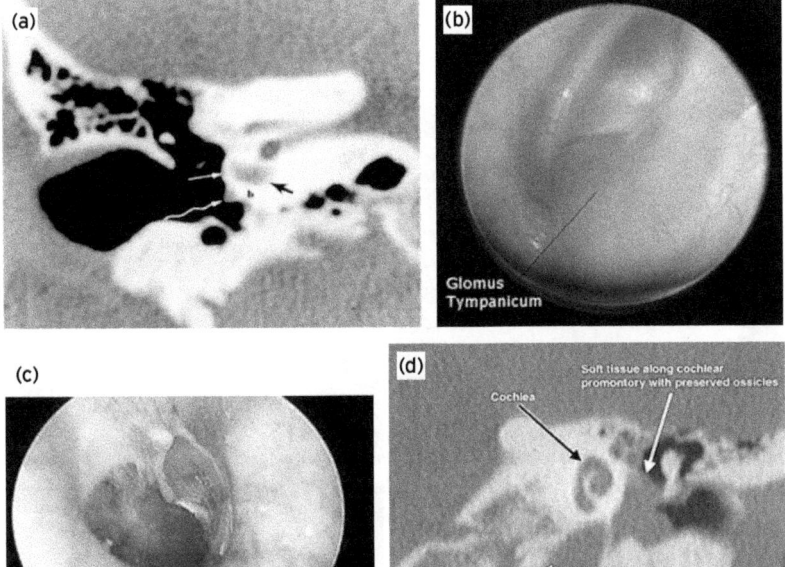

FIGURE 18-1 Glomus tympanic. (a) The otoscopic appearance of a glomus tympanicum.[13] (b) Tiny glomus tympanicum tumor. (a and b) Axial and coronal CT images in bone algorithm. (c and d) Axial and coronal, postcontrast-enhanced, T1-weighted images. The 2-mm glomus tympanicum tumor is located at the cochlear promontory, along the course of the inferior tympanic branch of the glossopharyngeal nerve (Jacobson nerve). It enhances following contrast administration (*arrow*).[14] (c) A pulsating red mass is seen behind the inferior half of the tympanic membrane.[15]

foramen, they readily (but not universally) cause lower CN palsies, either from tumor growth, or as a result of surgical excision. Vernet's syndrome is dysfunction of CNs IX, X, and XI. Villaret's syndrome is more extensive lower nerve dysfunction and includes CNs VII, IX, X, XI, and XII.

Classification systems have been developed to standardize reporting and treatment protocols and to anticipate related morbidity and mortality.[3] The Alford-Guilford system of the 1960s is not in clinical use.

The Glasscock-Jackson classification system is separated into GT and GJ.[4] The Glasscock-Jackson classification scheme for GT is as follows. Type I is GT limited to the promontory. Type II GTs completely fill the middle ear space. In type III, the GT fills the middle ear and extends to the

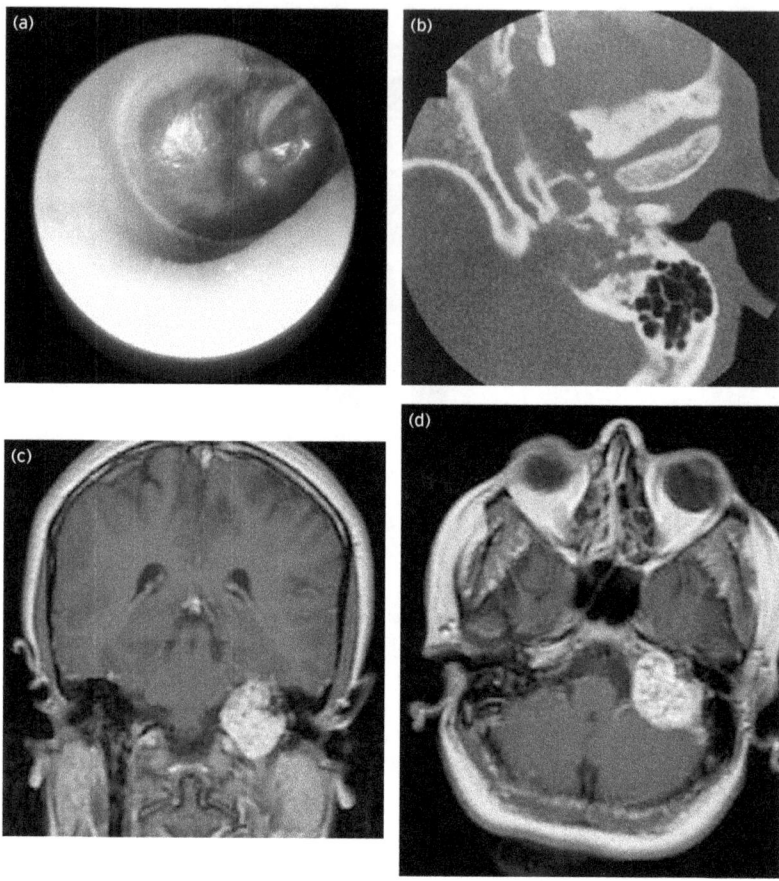

FIGURE 18-2 Glomus jugulare. (a) Otomicroscopic view of a tympanic glomangioma (inferior quadrant).[16] (b) Axial CT image of the temporal bone showing a right glomus jugulare tumor. Note the permeative destruction of bone (*arrow*) centered around the jugular bulb.[17] (c) Glomus jugulare tumor extending to involve the mastoid facial nerve. Axial CT images. (A) The expansile tumor causes moth-eaten destruction of the adjacent bone, centered at the jugular foramen. Note destruction of the petrous carotid canal (*arrow*). (b) More superiorly, involvement of the mastoid FNC is seen. Its medial margin has been eroded (*arrow*).[14] (d) T1-weighted magnetic resonance imaging scan with contrast showing a glomus tumor (T) occupying the right jugular fossa extending to the skull base. Note the internal carotid arteries (*arrows*).[18]

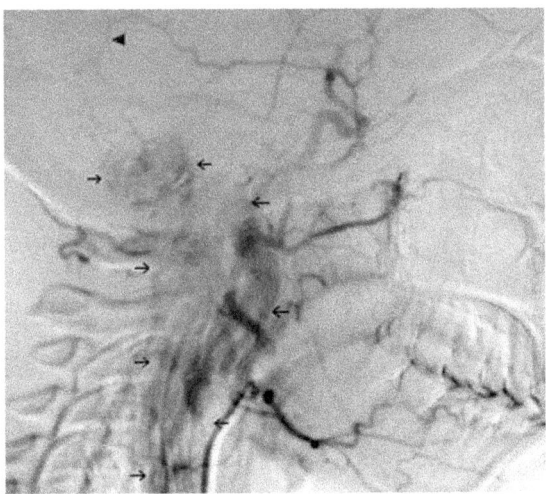

FIGURE 18-3 Left common carotid arteriogram of a patient with contralateral glomus jugulare demonstrating carotid body (*large arrow*) and glomus vagale (*small arrow*) tumors. The internal carotid artery is anteromedially displaced (*arrowhead*).[18]

mastoid. The largest GTs, type IV, extend into the external auditory canal and may extend anterior to the internal carotid artery.

The Glasscock-Jackson classification system for GJ is as follows. Type I involves the jugular bulb, middle ear, and mastoid. Types II–IV may have intracranial extension. Type II extends underneath the internal auditory canal. Type III GJs extend into the petrous apex. Type IV extends into the clivus and infratemporal fossa.

The Fisch Classification System[5] for all types of glomus tumors is as follows. Type A is limited to the middle ear cleft. Type B is limited to the tympanomastoid complex, and there is no infralabyrinthine involvement. Type C involves the labyrinth and extends to the petrous apex. In type D, there is intracranial involvement.

Fisch type C is further subdivided depending on the degree of invasion of the carotid canal as follows. Type C1 and C2 refer to limited and frank invasion, respectively, of the vertical portion of the carotid canal. Type C3 tumors have extension into the horizontal portion of the carotid canal. Fisch type D glomus tumors are subdivided into D1 and D2, by the degree of intracranial extension being either less than or greater than 2 cm.

GJ tumors are well-vascularized tumors and surgical management involves preoperative angiography and embolization, followed by mastoidectomy, upper cervical neck dissection with control of the great vessels, and management of the facial nerve, which runs directly through the surgical field.[6,7] Another treatment option for these tumors is external-beam radiation therapy, which can control tumor growth for up to 10–20 years,[8] or gamma knife radiosurgery, with marginal tumor doses of at least 13 Gy.[9]

One meta-analysis comparing GJ treatments (eight series of radiosurgery and seven series of surgery) found the following.[10] The mean age at treatment for patients who underwent surgery and radiosurgery was 47.3 and 56.7 years, respectively. The mean follow-up duration was 4 years for surgery and 3.25 years for radiation. The surgical control rate was 92.1%, with 88.2% of tumors totally resected in the initial surgery. A cerebrospinal fluid leak occurred in 8.3% of surgical patients; the mortality rate was 1.3%. For radiosurgery, tumors diminished in 36.5% and stayed the same size in 61.3%. Despite the presence of residual tumor in 100%, recurrences were found in only 2.1%, the morbidity rate was 8.5%, and there were no deaths.

Surgical extirpation with the goal of complete excision, with preoperative angiography and embolization to minimize intraoperative bleeding, is the treatment of choice in young patients.[11] Radiation therapy as an adjunct in the case of incomplete excision (usually because of CN concerns) is very effective.[12] Radiation alone is the treatment of choice in the older patient in whom surgery may be risky, because tumor control can last sufficiently in this age group.

The treating physician must address any lower CN palsies, particularly when there is concern regarding vocal fold weakness and lack of airway protection. Although out of the scope of this text, there are a number of voice therapy, procedural, and surgical interventions for these problems.

CASE HISTORY (PART 2)

This 37-year-old patient has a right GJ with lower CN involvement. If imaging indicates that there is no intracranial extension, surgical removal with preservation of facial nerve function is the correct treatment option. Preoperative angiography and embolization should be performed within

24–48 hours of the planned surgery. The primary risks of surgery are related to the CNs, but in this patient, the lower CNs are already paralyzed and therefore not at risk of new damage from surgery. Therefore, the real primary risk is to facial nerve function. This can usually be preserved with modification of surgical technique. If there is intracranial extension, a combined neurosurgical/neurotologic procedure is indicated. If the situation precludes complete tumor removal, radiation may be used for the residual tumor. Intervention for the lower CN palsies, particularly protection of the airway, can be done simultaneously.

> **KEY POINTS TO REMEMBER**
>
> - Paragangliomas may present with pulsatile tinnitus, conductive hearing loss, and/or lower cranial neuropathy.
> - CT of the temporal bone distinguishes between GT and GJ; magnetic resonance imaging is used to delineate extension of GJ tumors.
> - GT tumors are amenable to complete surgical excision.
> - GJ tumors may be treated with surgery, radiation, or both.

Further Reading
1. Weissman JL, Hirsch BE. Beyond the promontory: the multifocal origin of glomus tympanicum tumors. AJNR Am J Neuroradiol 1998;19:119–22.
2. Jackson CG, Welling DB, Chironis P, Glasscock ME III, Woods CI. Glomus tympanicum tumors: contemporary concepts in conservation surgery. Laryngoscope 1989;99:875–84.
3. Brackmann DE, Shelton C, Arriaga MA. Otologic Surgery, 3rd edition. Philadelphia: Saunders, 2010. pp. 551–67.
4. Jackson CG, Glasscock ME III, Harris PF. Glomus tumors. Diagnosis, classification, and management of large lesions. Arch Otolaryngol 1982;108:401–10.
5. Fisch U, Mattox D. Microsurgery of the Skull Base. New York: Thieme, 1988. pp. 149–220.
6. Leonetti JP, Anderson DE, Marzo SJ, Origitano TC, Vandevender D, Quinonez R. Facial paralysis associated with glomus jugulare tumors. Otol Neurotol 2007;28:104–6.
7. Jackson CG. Glomus tympanicum and glomus jugulare tumors. Otolaryngol Clin North Am 2001;34:941–70, vii.
8. Brackmann DE, House WF, Terry R, Scanlan RL. Glomus jugulare tumors: effect of irradiation. Trans Am Acad Ophthalmol Otolaryngol 1972;76:1423–31.

9. Chen PG, Nguyen JH, Payne SC, Sheehan JP, Hashisaki GT. Treatment of glomus jugulare tumors with gamma knife radiosurgery. Laryngoscope 2010;120:1856–62.
10. Gottfried ON, Liu JK, Couldwell WT. Comparison of radiosurgery and conventional surgery for the treatment of glomus jugulare tumors. Neurosurg Focus 2004;17:E4.
11. Green JD Jr, Brackmann DE, Nguyen CD, Arriaga MA, Telischi FF, De la Cruz A. Surgical management of previously untreated glomus jugulare tumors. Laryngoscope 1994;104(8 Pt 1):917–21.
12. Fayad JN, Keles B, Brackmann DE. Jugular foramen tumors: clinical characteristics and treatment outcomes. Otol Neurotol 2010;31:299–305.
13. Dhillon RS, East CA (Eds.). FRCS - Ear, Nose and Throat and Head and Neck Surgery. Churchill Livingstone Elsevier, Philadelphia, PA. 2013. pp. 87–117.
14. Julaino, Tsang, AF. Temporal bone tumors and cerebellopontine angle lesions. In: P Som, H Curtin (Eds.). Head and Neck Imaging. Mosby, 2011. Marceline, Missouri. pp. 1263–407.
15. Ying-Liang C. En bloc surgical removal of an asymptomatic glomus tympanicum tumor. J Chinese Med Assoc 2011;74:520–2.
16. Massimo G. Glomus tumors. In: Winn HR (Ed.). Youmans Neurological Surgery. Saunders, Philadelphia, PA. 2011. pp. 1594–609.
17. St. Martin MB. Imaging of hearing loss. Otolaryngol Clin North Am 2008;41:157–78.
18. Hirsch BE. Glomus tumors. In: Myers EN (Ed.). Operative Otolaryngology: Head and Neck Surgery. Saunders, Philadelphia, PA. 2008. pp. 1319–35.

19 Arteriovenous Malformations, Arteriovenous Fistulas, and Aberrant Vasculature

A 30-year-old man presents with unilateral pulsatile tinnitus of several months' duration. He denies hearing loss. He has intermittent headaches and mild lightheadedness, which occurs infrequently. He denies vision disturbance. He denies history of head trauma and ear surgery. Physical examination is negative for ear, nose, throat, or head and neck abnormalities. Ophthalmologic examination is normal.

What do you do now?

ARTERIOVENOUS MALFORMATIONS

Arteriovenous malformations (AVM) of the temporal bone are often associated with the presentation of pulsatile tinnitus. An AVM is a vascular abnormality constituted by a complex, tangled web of afferent arteries and draining veins linked by an abnormal dysplastic intervening capillary bed.

Cerebral AVMs occur at about one-tenth the frequency of aneurysms, at an adult point prevalence of approximately 18 per 100,000. The detection rate for symptomatic AVMs is 0.8%–0.14% per year. In about half the patients with AVMs, the first symptoms are those of a stroke caused by bleeding into the brain. A total of 10% of those cases end in death. Symptoms of an AVM that has not bled include pulsatile tinnitus; confusion; headache; seizures; and symptoms of increased intracerebral pressure, such as vision changes, dizziness, muscle weakness, and paresthesias. AVMs that do not cause symptoms by the late 40s or early 50s will most likely never cause symptoms.[1,2] There is a Spetzler-Marlin grading system for cerebral AVMs; this is not pertinent for management of tinnitus per se.

Temporal bone AVMs are a small subset of cerebral AVMs. Diagnosis is made by imaging. The management of AVM of the temporal bone can be challenging. Although microsurgery and radiosurgery can be of benefit for other AVM symptoms, it is not clear whether AVM-related tinnitus can be resolved with these types of interventions.

Imaging of AVMs is performed with computed tomography (CT) scan, which can identify intracerebral hemorrhage and raise suspicion of a small AVM or identify a large AVM, and magnetic resonance imaging, which is essential for the initial diagnosis of AVM (Figure 19-1).[3] Conventional or magnetic resonance angiography delineates the AVM clearly (Figure 19-2).

Since the 1980s, progressive advances in preoperative embolization, frameless stereotaxy, and intraoperative electrophysiologic monitoring have significantly increased the number of posterior fossa AVMs that are amenable to microsurgical resection with minimal morbidity and mortality.[4] However, there are case reports of transient facial and trigeminal neuropathies resulting from embolization of skull base AVMs.[5]

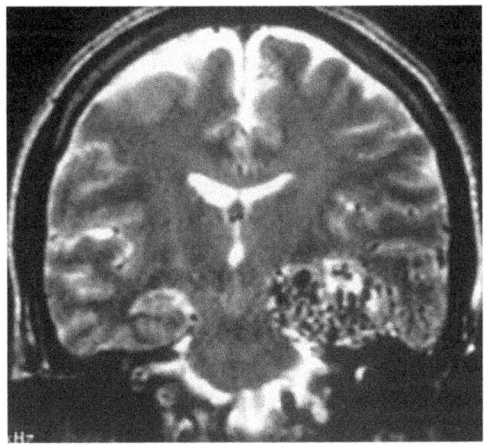

FIGURE 19-1 Magnetic resonance image and computed tomography of temporal lobe arteriovenous malformation. T2 coronal magnetic resonance image showing an arteriovenous malformation in the left medial temporal lobe.[15] Computed tomography angiography showed an arteriovenous malformation in the left temporal lobe, which was confirmed by magnetic resonance imaging. Angiography and especially three-dimensional digital subtraction angiography outlined the posterior communicating and anterior choroidal arteries as feeders.

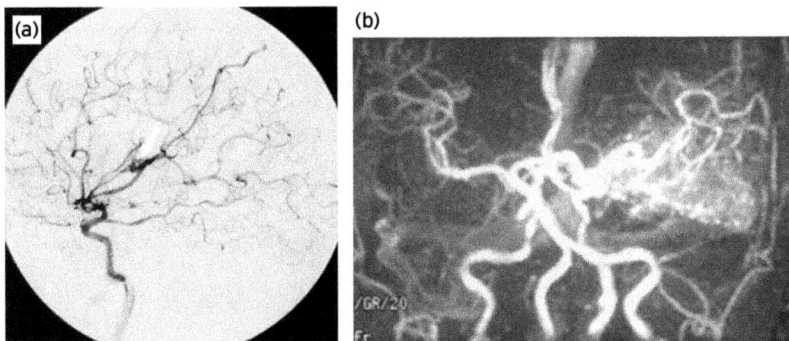

FIGURE 19-2 Angiogram of right temporal arteriovenous malformations. (a) Lateral common carotid injection demonstrates prompt filling of the vertebral artery from muscular collaterals of the occipital artery. The anterior circulation fills via the posterior communicating artery in this patient with occlusive disease of the internal carotid artery. (Source: Johnson et al. Vascular anatomy of the head, neck, and skull base. In: Hurst RW, Rosenwasser RH, editors. Interventional Neuroradiology. New York: Taylor and Frances, 2007; with permission.) (b) Selective occipital arteriography demonstrates enlarged dural branches of the OCC with fistulization (*arrows*) to the transverse sinus and shunting into the sinus and jugular vein in this patient with dural arteriovenous malformations and tinnitus.[16]

ARTERIOVENOUS FISTULAS

Unlike an AVM, an arteriovenous fistula (AVF) has direct fistulous connection without the intervening nidus of dysplastic capillaries. Dural AVFs (Figure 19-3) present with pulsatile tinnitus and headache, papilledema, proptosis, blepharoptosis, visual changes, and hemiparesis. Although the true incidence of intracranial dural AVF is not known, they seem to occur one-tenth as frequently as intracerebral AVMs. Many dural AVFs remain clinically silent or involute spontaneously.

Treatments include surgery, interventional angiography, and radiation. There is demonstrated use of arterial ligation for dural AVF.[6] Endovascular treatment by either arterial (preferentially) or venous route can be

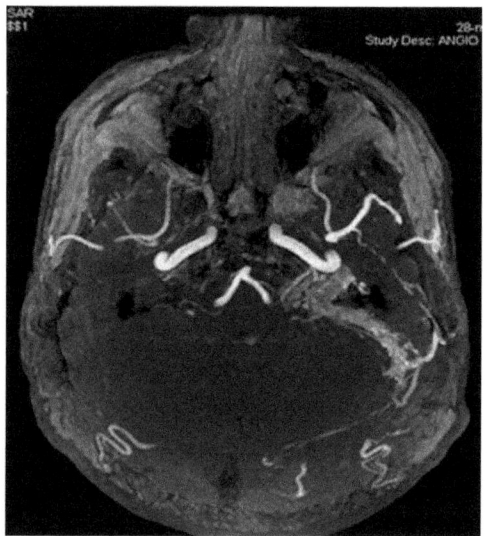

FIGURE 19-3 Magnetic resonance image of arteriovenous fistula. A 51-year-old man with constant left pulsatile tinnitus, noted to progressively worsen over the past 6-month period, and negative noninvasive imaging workup including magnetic resonance imaging and magnetic resonance angiography and skull base computed tomography. DSA, left common carotid injection, anteroposterior view, obtained during diagnostic angiography (June 23, 2011). A left transverse sinus Dural arteriovenous fistula is documented, principally fed by multiple branches of the left occipital artery, with purely antegrade drainage into the left internal jugular vein (Merland-Cognard type I). DSA, left common carotid injection, anteroposterior view, obtained at the beginning of the therapeutic procedure performed 1 month later (July 25, 2011). Retrograde drainage into the right transverse sinus and right internal jugular vein is now observed (Merland-Cognard type IIa). (Courtesy of Phillipe Gailloud.)

successful in ameliorating the tinnitus.[7] Occasionally, radiosurgery is indicated. Aggressive management of AVF solely for the treatment of pulsatile tinnitus presents significant risks, and should be considered deliberately in a multidisciplinary manner before being pursued.[8]

A rare, usually posttraumatic AVF is carotid-cavernous fistula (CCF), which is a communication between the internal or external carotid artery and the cavernous sinus.[9] A total of 75% are direct CCFs between the intracavernous segment of the internal carotid artery and the cavernous sinus. They have high rates of arterial blood flow and are commonly caused by a single traumatic tear in the arterial wall. The 25% that are dural CCFs may represent congenital AVMs, have low rates of arterial blood flow, and are "spontaneous" without antecedent trauma. Those occur in middle-aged to elderly women with or without underlying vascular or connective tissue disease. Unlike the patient presentation above, CCFs present with significant ophthalmologic findings, including proptosis and pulsating exophthalmos. Diagnosis is made by CT scan, magnetic resonance imaging, orbital echography, and cerebral arteriography. Treatment is directed to eye protection and vision recovery, and CCF treatment is surgical or endovascular in nature.[10]

ABERRANT VASCULATURE

Jugular bulb anomalies (JBA) (Figure 19-4) are often associated with pulsatile tinnitus. A review of 30 JBA identified on CT scan and 1,579 temporal bone specimens[11] revealed that 50% of the patients with JBA were asymptomatic. Symptoms may include pulsatile tinnitus, vertigo, or conductive hearing loss. The natural history of JBA is not known. Another review of 52 cases of high jugular bulb reveals the following.[12] Most people with high jugular bulb remain asymptomatic. As with JBA, the best diagnostic tool is high-resolution CT scan. There are case reports of successful jugular vein ligation in patients with high jugular bulb with intractable pulsatile tinnitus; however, there are also reports that ligation and/or compression of the jugular vein and sigmoid sinus is not beneficial.[13] At the least, the patient should be tested in the office with ipsilateral compression of the jugular vein to determine if that resolves the pulsatile tinnitus before considering surgery or other intervention.

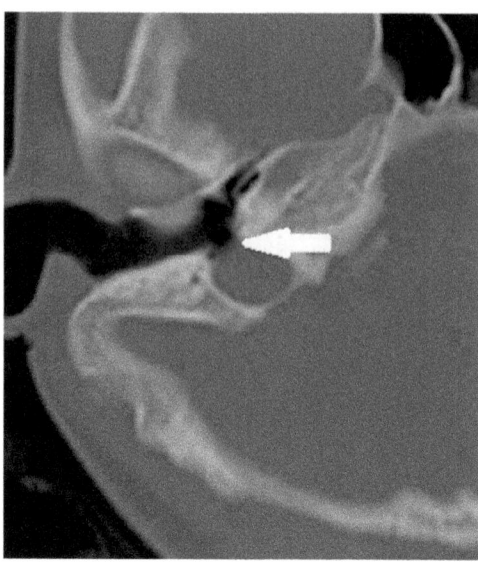

FIGURE 19-4 Dehiscent jugular bulb with a diverticulum. Contrast-enhanced computed tomography temporal bones show a dehiscent and high-riding jugular bulb (*arrow*) with a diverticulum into the right middle ear cavity (*asterisk*). Coronal reformat image through temporal bones shows the dehiscent jugular bulb (*arrow*) with small diverticulum (*asterisk*).[17]

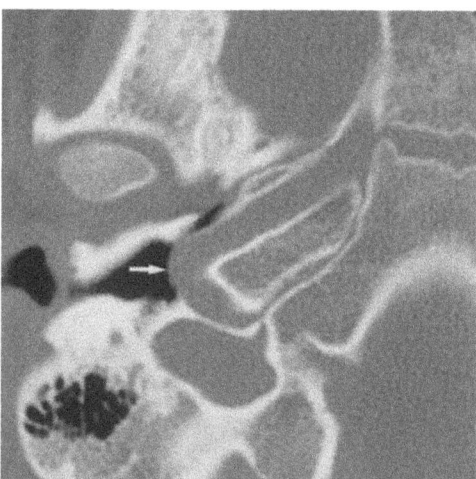

FIGURE 19-5 Aberrant internal carotid artery. Preoperative (axial; coronal) and postoperative (axial; coronal) computed tomography images of the aberrant internal carotid artery (ICA). An aberrant course of the right ICA was demonstrated through a dehiscent lateral carotid plate (*arrows*). The tympanic membrane made contact with the ICA (*arrowheads*). After the operation, there was enough space between ICA (*arrows*) and tympanic membrane (*arrowheads*).[18]

Aberrant internal carotid artery in the middle ear is an exceptionally rare, potential cause of pulsatile tinnitus. CT scan makes the diagnosis (Figure 19-5). Magnetic resonance imaging and magnetic resonance angiography may further elucidate this rare situation. In a review of 86 cases of aberrant internal carotid artery, hearing loss was present in 41 and pulsatile tinnitus in 26 cases. Inadvertent injury to an aberrant internal carotid artery may result in brisk bleeding, hemiparesis, aphasia, deafness, Horner syndrome, and intractable vertigo. In general, conservative management with yearly follow-up is indicated.[14]

> **KEY POINTS TO REMEMBER**
>
> - Temporal bone AVMs occur infrequently, and can be addressed with microsurgery or radiosurgery; however, treatment of AVMs may not resolve the symptoms of pulsatile tinnitus.
> - AVFs are rare and are usually amenable to endovascular treatment, which can ameliorate the symptom of pulsatile tinnitus.
> - CCF is a rare, often posttraumatic, type of AVF. Treatment for this is either surgical or endovascular.
> - High-riding jugular bulb is not an uncommon finding; jugular vein ligation in those patients may or may not resolve their pulsatile tinnitus.

Further Reading
1. Selman WR, Blackham K, Tarr RW, Ratcheson RA. Vascular diseases of the nervous system: vascular malformations. In: Bradley WG, Daroff RB, Fenichel GM, Jankovic J, editors. Bradley: Neurology in Clinical Practice, 5th edition. Philadelphia: Butterworth Heinemann Elsevier, 2008.
2. Laakso A, Dashti R, Juvela S, Niemelä M, Hernesniemi J. Natural history of arteriovenous malformations: presentation, risk of hemorrhage and mortality. Acta Neurochir Suppl 2010;107:65–9.
3. Weissman JL, Hirsch BE. Imaging of tinnitus: a review. Radiology 2000;216:342–9.
4. Sinclair J, Kelly ME, Steinberg GK. Surgical management of posterior fossa arteriovenous malformations. Neurosurgery 2006;58:ONS-189–ONS-201.
5. Nyberg EM, Chaudry MI, Turk AS, Turner RD. Transient cranial neuropathies as sequelae of onyx embolization of arteriovenous shunt lesions near the skull base: possible axonotmetic traction injuries. J Neurointervent Surg 2013;5:e21.

6. Courteney-Harris RG, Ford GR, Innes AJ, Colin JF. Pulsatile tinnitus: three cases of arteriovenous fistula treated by ligation of the occipital artery. J Laryngol Otol 1990;104:421–2.
7. Delgado F, Munoz F, Bravo-Rodriguez F, Jurado-Ramos A, Oteros R. Treatment of dural arteriovenous fistulas presenting as pulsatile tinnitus. Otol Neurotol 2009;30:897–902.
8. Adams W, Whitfield P. Intracranial dural arteriovenous fistulae. Advances in Clinical Neuroscience and Rehabilitation 2007;7.
9. Debrun GM, Vinuela F, Fox AJ, et al. Indications for treatment and classification of 132 carotid-cavernous fistulas. Neurosurgery 1988;22:285–9.
10. Kirsch M, Henkes H, Liebig T, et al. Endovascular management of dural carotid-cavernous sinus fistulas in 141 patients. Neuroradiology 2006;48:486–90.
11. Friedmann DR, Eubig J, Winata LS, Pramanik BK, Merchant SN, Lalwani AK. A clinical and histopathologic study of jugular bulb abnormalities. Arch Otolaryngol Head Neck Surg 2012;138:66–71.
12. Lin DJ, Hsu CJ, Lin KN. The high jugular bulb: report of five cases and a review of the literature. J Formos Med Assoc 1993;92:745–50.
13. Jackler RK, Brackmann DE, Sismanis A. A warning on venous ligation for pulsatile tinnitus. Otol Neurotol 2001;22:427–8.
14. Windfuhr JP. Aberrant internal carotid artery in the middle ear. Ann Otol Rhinol Laryngol Suppl 2004;192:1–16.
15. Mueller-Kronast N. Vascular anomalies of the brain. In: Rabinstein A, Resnick SJ (Eds.). Practical Neuroimaging in Stroke. Saunders, Philadelphia, PA. 2009. pp. 321–69.
16. Michele H. Johnson, Hjalti M. Thorisson, Michael L. DiLuna. Vascular anatomy: the head, neck, and skull base. Neurosurg Clin North Am 20(3):239-258.
17. Kang M. Imaging of tinnitus. Otolaryngol Clin North Am 2008;41:179–93.
18. Honkura Y, Hidaka H, Ohta J, Gorai S, Ka1tori Y, Kobayashi T. Surgical treatment for the aberrant internal carotid artery in the middle ear with pulsatile tinnitus. Auris Nasus Larynx. 2014;41(2):215-8.

20 Benign Intracranial Hypertension

A 30-year-old woman presents with pulsatile tinnitus of several months' duration. She denies hearing loss. She has intermittent headaches and mild lightheadedness. She has occasionally blurry vision. She denies history of head trauma or ear surgery. Physical examination is significant for a moderately obese female in no acute distress and is negative for ear, nose, throat, or head and neck abnormalities. Ophthalmologic examination reveals papilledema. There are no audible bruits or palpable thrills. Audiogram is normal. Lumbar puncture shows increased intracranial pressure, and alleviates patient's tinnitus complaints.

What do you do now?

Benign intracranial hypertension (BIH), also called idiopathic intracranial hypertension and pseudotumor cerebri, should be considered a clinical emergency until the presence or absence of an underlying intracranial mass is confirmed by neuroimaging. The modified Dandy diagnostic criteria for BIH include (1) signs and symptoms of intracranial pressure, (2) no localizing neurologic signs other than unilateral or bilateral sixth nerve palsies, (3) increased cerebrospinal fluid (CSF) pressures without

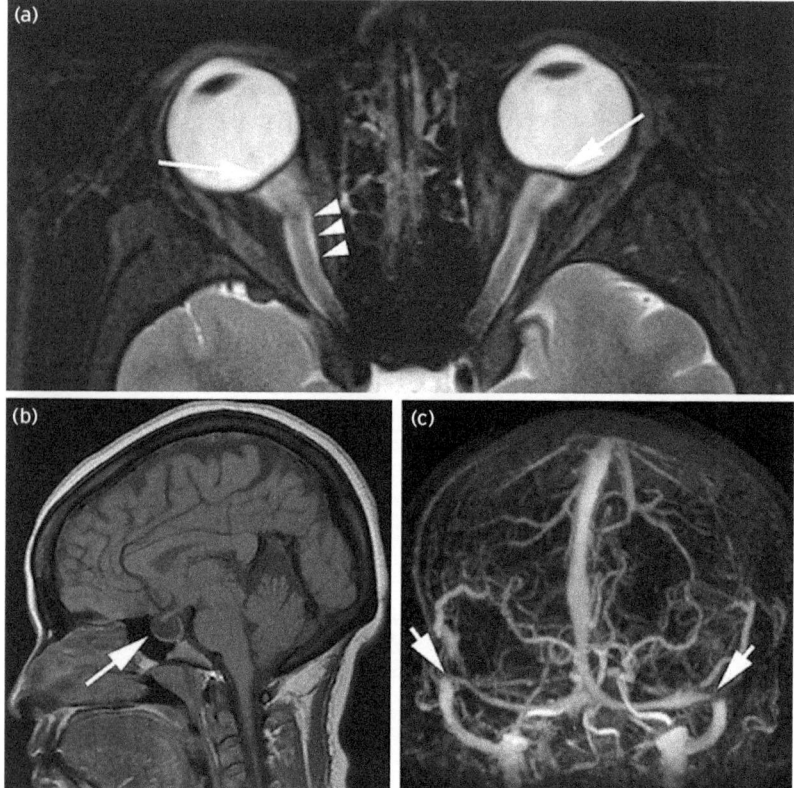

FIGURE 20-1 (a) Magnetic resonance imaging venogram and magnetic resonance imaging findings associated with pseudotumor cerebri. Empty sella (*open white arrow*) is demonstrated in sagittal T1-weighted image. Note the absence of the normal pituitary contents, which seem pushed to the bottom of the sella.[4] (b) Magnetic resonance venogram showing smooth-walled venous stenoses of the transverse sinus, characteristic of idiopathic intracranial hypertension.[5] (c) T2-weighted image shows optic disc elevation (*black arrows*), dilated optic nerve sheaths (*white arrows*), tortuous optic nerves, and indentation of the globes posteriorly.[4]

other CSF abnormalities, and (4) presence of normal-to-small symmetric ventricles. Additional criteria are as follows: diagnostic lumbar puncture should be done with the patient in the lateral decubitus position, magnetic resonance imaging or magnetic resonance venography should be done to rule out intracranial venous sinus stenosis or thrombosis, and other causes of intracranial hypertension are ruled out.[1]

BIH occurs in 0.9 per 100,000 general population, but 13–14.85 per 100,000 in women aged 20–44 years and 10% over their ideal weight, and 19.3 per 100,000 in women 20% above their ideal weight. In individuals 38% over their ideal weight, there is an 8:1 female/male ratio of BIH.

Although it is common in overweight women and weight loss seems to help the symptoms, the role that obesity plays in BIH is unclear. Magnetic resonance imaging findings in BIH include optic nerve and globe abnormalities, empty sella, and transverse sinus stenosis (Figure 20-1). The prolonged remission of symptoms that follows removal of CSF via lumbar puncture is presumably caused by relief of the 40% venous sinus (usually transverse sinus) stenosis that is seen in these patients. BIH is treated with weight loss, including and up to bariatric surgery, diuretics, headache prophylaxis, and corticosteroids for flare-ups of symptoms. These measures often provide pulsatile tinnitus resolution.[2]

If BIH is not treated appropriately, irreversible optic neuropathy may develop. Rarely, and only for life-threatening and vision-threatening BIH, the patient may require optic nerve sheath fenestration, CSF diversion procedures (e.g., lumboperitoneal shunt), or intracranial venous sinus stenting. These procedures are not done for pulsatile tinnitus alone.[3]

> **KEY POINTS TO REMEMBER**
>
> - Diagnostic criteria for BIH include signs and symptoms of increased intracranial pressure, either no localizing neurologic signs or sixth nerve palsy only, increased CSF pressure, and normal ventricles.
> - BIH is more common in women and in overweight and obese patients.
> - Lumbar puncture may be therapeutic.
> - Other treatments for pulsatile tinnitus in BIH include weight loss, diuretics, headache prophylaxis, and short courses of corticosteroids for flare-ups.

Further Reading

1. Friedman DI, Jacobson DM. Diagnostic criteria for idiopathic intracranial hypertension. Neurology 2002;59:1492–5.
2. Michaelides EM, Sismanis A, Sugerman HJ, Felton WL III. Pulsatile tinnitus in patients with morbid obesity: the effectiveness of weight reduction surgery. Am J Otol 2000;21:682–5.
3. Jindal M, Hiam L, Raman A, Rejali D. Idiopathic intracranial hypertension in otolaryngology. Eur Arch Otorhinolaryngol 2009;266:803–6.
4. Liu GT. Optic disc swelling: papilledema and other causes. In: Neuro-Ophthalmology: Diagnosis and Management. Saunders, Elsevier, Philadelphia, PA. 2010. pp. 199–236.
5. Wall M. Idiopathic intracranial hypertension. Neurol Clin 2010;28:593–617.

21 Tegmen Dehiscence, Including Superior Semicircular Canal Dehiscence

A 42-year-old woman presents with right-sided pulsatile tinnitus of several months' duration. She notes hearing loss in the right ear since her mastoidectomy surgery for cholesteatoma 20 years ago. She has rare right-sided headaches. She denies vertigo or blurry vision. Physical examination is significant for a moderately obese female in no acute distress. Ear, nose, throat, and head and neck examination is significant for right canal wall up mastoidectomy with no evidence of active cholesteatoma or chronic otitis media. Tuning fork examination indicates right conductive hearing loss. Ophthalmologic examination is negative. There are no audible bruits or palpable thrills. Audiogram shows right mixed hearing loss, primarily conductive, with good word recognition ability.

What do you do now?

Tegmen dehiscence (TD) is unusual without a history of prior ear surgery but is seen after remote mastoid surgery, and it is a possibility in the workup of pulsatile tinnitus. TD has been reported in children without prior significant ear history treated for acute mastoiditis.[1] Diagnosis is made by axial and coronal computed tomography (CT) scan of the temporal bones, which demonstrates the bony dehiscence and often the associated encephalocoele (Figure 21-1). Treatment includes transmastoid reduction of the encephalocoele and repair of the tegmen defect.[2]

Superior semicircular canal dehiscence (SSCD) is thinning or absence of the otic capsule bone over the SSC. It was first described by Lloyd Minor in 2000.[3] There is evidence that SSCD begins with developmental defects of the tegmen, with small series of patients with multiple TD and SSCD, without history of prior ear surgery.[4,5] Histopathologic examination of the temporal bone of a patient with, among other symptoms, pulsatile tinnitus showed a frank right SSCD, thin bone over the left SSC, and focal microdehiscences of the tegmen bilaterally.[6] This confirms the hypothesis of failure of postnatal bone development with minor trauma disrupting thin bone or previously stable dura over the SSC. A radiologic review of CT findings in 38 patients with SSCD compared with 41 control subjects showed a 10.2 times higher odds of having radiographic TD in either ear for the patients with SSCD. Additionally, the larger the width of the SSCD, the higher the relative risk for TD, up to more than two-fold (Figure 21-2).[7]

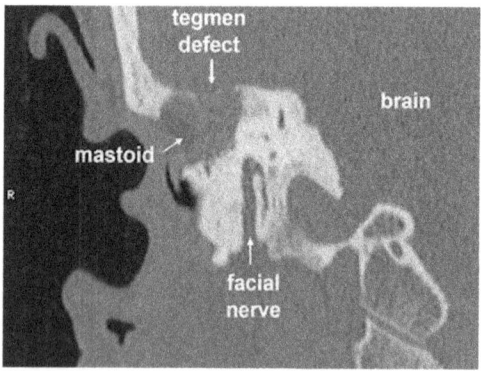

FIGURE 21-1 Tegmen dehiscence with meningoencephalocele. High-resolution CT scan (coronal view) of the right temporal bone. Dehiscence of the tegmen tympani with meningoencephalocele.[8]

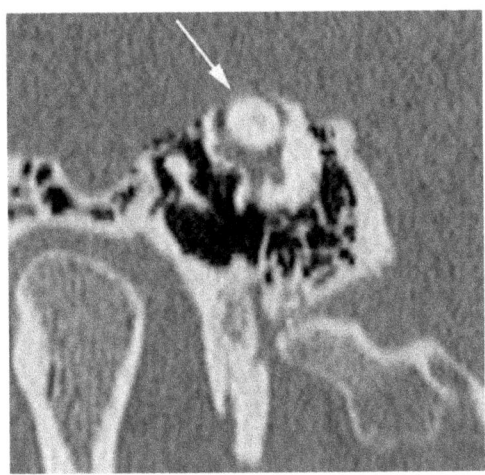

FIGURE 21-2 Tegmen dehiscence with meningoencephalocele. High-resolution CT scan (coronal view) reveals a dehiscence in both tegmen tympani and superior semicircular canal in left and right temporal bone.[8] Sagittal oblique noncontrast CT scan showing large SSCD and dehiscence of tegmen antrii over ossicles.[9] Reformatted high-resolution, noncontrast, coronal temporal bone CT scans of a patient who had undergone prior right stapedotomy for presumed otosclerosis (case 1). The study shows a dehiscent superior semicircular canal on the right (*white arrow*) and left (*white arrowhead*). The stapes prosthesis is shown within the vestibule on the right (*black arrow*). Normal left vestibule (*black double arrow*) is shown for comparison.[10]

KEY POINTS TO REMEMBER

- TD is usually seen in the setting of a history of prior ear surgery.
- TD may be seen in children with a prior history of acute mastoiditis but without a history of prior ear surgery.
- SSCD is suspected in patients with dizziness disorders, ipsilateral tinnitus, suprathreshold bone conduction on audiogram, and abnormal vestibular evoked myogenic potential. Additionally, a tuning fork placed on the ipsilateral lateral malleolus of the ankle may be perceived in the ear with SSCD.
- SSCD is diagnosed by targeted temporal bone CT scans obtained in the sagittal plane.

Further Reading
1. Mallur PS, Harirchian S, Lalwani AK. Preoperative and postoperative intracranial complications of acute mastoiditis. Ann Otol Rhinol Laryngol 2009;118:118–23.
2. Kale SU, Pfleiderer AG, Cradwick JC. Bilateral defects of the tegmen tympani associated with brain and dural prolapse in a patient with pulsatile tinnitus. J Laryngol Otol 2000;114:861–3.
3. Minor LB. Superior canal dehiscence syndrome. Am J Otol 2000;21:9–19.
4. Suryanarayanan R, Lesser TH. "Honeycomb" tegmen: multiple tegmen defects associated with superior semicircular canal dehiscence. J Laryngol Otol 2010;124:560–3.
5. Mahendran S, Sunkaraneni VS, Baguley DM, Axon PR. Superior semicircular canal dehiscence with a large tegmental defect. J Laryngol Otol 2007;121:189–91.
6. Teixido M, Kung B, Rosowski JJ, Merchant SN. Histopathology of the temporal bone in a case of superior canal dehiscence syndrome. Ann Otol Rhinol Laryngol 2012;121:7–12.
7. Nadaraja GS, Gurgel RK, Fischbein NJ, et al. Radiographic evaluation of the tegmen in patients with superior semicircular canal dehiscence. Otol Neurotol 2012;33:1245–50. doi:10.1097/MAO.0b013e3182634e27.
8. Markou K. Spontaneous osteodural defects of the temporal bone: diagnosis and management of 12 cases. Am J Otolaryngol Head Neck Med Surg 2011;32:135–40.
9. Lane JI, Lindell P, Witte RJ, DeLone DR, Driscoll CLW. Middle and inner ear: improved depiction with multiplanar reconstruction of volumetric CT data. Radiographics 2006;26:115–24.
10. Li PMMC. Superior semicircular canal dehiscence diagnosed after failed stapedotomy for conductive hearing loss. Am J Otolaryngol Head Neck Med Surg 32:441–4.

SECTION IV

Facial Neuropathy

22 Congenital Facial Palsy

The general pediatrics service was consulted to evaluate a 1-day-old female neonate presented with findings of right-sided facial paresis. She was the first born to a 28-year-old healthy female. The pregnancy was uncomplicated. Appropriate prenatal care was received. She was born at 39 weeks gestation via vaginal delivery with forceps assistance secondary to prolonged stage two of delivery. Her Apgar scores were 6 at 1 minute and 9 at 5 minutes. The patient since delivery has been noted to have difficulty with latching on for feeding. The lactation consultant evaluated the patient and noted weak suckling. The mother expressed great concern at the fact that the infant is noted to have gross calvarial deformity and asymmetric facial motion during crying. On examination, the patient was a 9-pound 3-ounce female. She is appropriately developed. The remainder of the examination was within normal limits with the exception of an ecchymosis noted at the right mastoid tip and significant right facial paresis in the regions supplied by all branches of the facial nerve.

What do you do know?

Congenital facial palsy is a relatively uncommon occurrence. The estimated incidence of congenital facial palsy is approximately 0.8–2.1 per 1,000 births. In most (80%) patients born with congenital facial palsy, birth trauma is the etiology. Of patients who sustained birth trauma, 67%–91% underwent forceps-assisted delivery.[1-3] As such, forceps-assisted delivery is a risk factor for congenital traumatic facial palsy. In cases of birth trauma, the facial palsy more commonly is associated with a compression injury to the facial nerve as it exits the skull base. Within the normal neonate, the mastoid air cells and mastoid tips are underdeveloped. The mastoid and mastoid tip serves as a protection for the vertical segment of the facial nerve. Because of the lack of protection in this region along with the positioning of the forceps, compression and neuropraxia (Table 22-1) or first-degree injury to the nerve may occur.[4-6]

These patients typically present with hypofunction in all branches of the extratemporal facial nerve (Table 22-2) manifesting as asymmetry in all

TABLE 22-1 **Classification of Nerve Injury**

Sunderland Classification*	Seddon Classification	Description of Nerve Injury
I	Neuropraxia	Nerve conduction blockage (blockage of axoplasm flow within the axon, nerve conduction block), the action potential cannot be propagated across the site of lesion but a stimulation distal to the site of lesion yields a normal evoked response
II	Axonotmesis	Axonal and myelin disruption distal to the site of lesion resulting from progression of a first-degree injury representing wallerian degeneration
III		Complete disruption of the axon including its surrounding myelin and endoneurium
IV		Complete disruption of the perineurium
V		Complete disruption of the epineurium
VI	Neurotmesis	An addition to the traditional Sunderland classification characterized by normal function through some fascicles and varying degree of injury

*Described as degrees of injury.

TABLE 22-2 **Branches of the Facial Nerve**

Location of Branching	Branch	Function
Cerebellopontine angle	Nervus intermedius (Wrisberg nerve)	Rather than branching from, this nerve joins the facial nerve at the cerebellopontine angle; it mediate the functions of taste, cutaneous sensation of the external ear, proprioception, lacrimation, and salivation (submandibular, sublingual, and minor salivary glands)
Intratemporal	Greater superficial petrosal nerve	Taste sensation to the palate; parasympathetic supply to the lacrimal gland and mucosal glands of the nose, palate, and pharynx
	Chorda tympani	Taste sensation to the anterior two-thirds of the tongue
	Nerve to the stapedius	Innervation to the stapedius muscle
Extratemporal	Nerve to the stylohyoid	Innervation to the stylohoid muscle
	Temporal branch (frontal branch)	Innervation to the muscles of facial expression
	Zygomatic branch	Innervation to the muscles of facial expression
	Buccal branch	Innervation to the muscles of facial expression
	Marginal mandibular branch	Innervation to the muscles of facial expression
	Cervical branch	Innervation to the platysma

muscles of facial expression representing all branches of the extratemporal facial nerve. A history of difficulties during labor or forceps-assisted delivery should increase one's suspicion regarding trauma as a potential etiology. Additionally, clinical findings on examination that may increase the index of suspicion regarding birth trauma as the etiologic factor in congenital

TABLE 22-3 Nontraumatic Etiology of Congenital Facial Palsy

Classification	Etiologies	Characteristic Findings
Nonsyndromic	Congenital unilateral lower lip palsy	Palsy of the lower lip
	Familial congenital facial palsy	Unilateral facial palsy
Teratogens	Intrauterine thalidomide exposure	Facial and abducens nerve palsy, ear anomalies, phocomelia (reduction in the length of the long bones of the arms or legs)
	Intraunterine misoprostol exposure	Bilateral facial nerve palsy, unilateral or bilateral abducens nerve palsy, extremity abnormalities
Syndromic	Möbius syndrome	Bilateral facial nerve palsy, unilateral or bilateral abducens nerve palsy, extremity abnormalities
	Facioscapulohumeral muscular dystrophy	Distal myopathy including weakness of the face, jaw, neck, and levator palpebrae; facial diplegia with intact lateral gaze
	CHARGE syndrome	Colobomata, heart disease, choanal atresia, retarted growth, genital hypoplasia, ear anomalies, multiple cranial nerve palsies including facial nerve palsy
	22q11.2 deletion syndrome	Facial nerve palsy, congenital heart disease,
	Albers-Schönberg disease	Osteopetrosis, facial nerve palsy
	Hemifacial microsomia	Facial palsy, hearing loss (conductive or sensorineural), craniofacial deformity including first and second brachial arch derivatives
	Goldenhar syndrome	Facial palsy, hearing loss (conductive or sensorineural), craniofacial deformity including first and second brachial arch derivatives, vertebral anomalies, epibulbar dermoids

facial palsy include periauricular ecchymosis and hemotympanum. Facial palsy typically presents with progressive onset. In most patients (>90%), facial palsy resolves spontaneously.[7,8] For patients in whom spontaneous recovery does not occur radiographic and electrophysiologic evaluation should be used.[8-10] Eye protection including lubrication is mandatory to prevent damage to the cornea.

In patients without a history of birth trauma or forceps-assisted delivery, additional etiologies should be considered within the differential diagnosis when evaluating a neonate with congenital facial palsy. Nontraumatic congenital facial palsy may occur in both syndromic and nonsyndromic forms. Table 22-3 provides a list of potential nontraumatic etiologies of congenital facial palsy. The most commonly encountered nontraumatic etiology of congenital facial palsy is congenital unilateral lower lip paralysis. Of note, congenital unilateral lower lip paralysis is not associated with hypofunction of the facial nerve, but rather hypoplasia or congenital absence of the depressor anularis oris or depressor labii inferioris muscles. These patients tend to have associated cardiac anomalies, so cardiac evaluation is warranted.

Patients presenting with nontraumatic etiology of congenital facial palsy should be screened on physical examination for the associated findings listed in Table 22-3. If physical findings increase the clinical index of suspicion regarding possible syndromic association, a genetics consultation should be obtained.

> **KEY POINTS TO REMEMBER**
>
> - Congenital facial palsy is relatively uncommon
> - The most common cause of congenital facial palsy is birth trauma typically involving forceps delivery
> - The most common nontraumatic cause of facial palsy is congenital unilateral lower lip paralysis

Further Reading

1. Falco NA, Eriksson E. Facial nerve palsy in the newborn: incidence and outcome. Plast Reconstr Surg 1990;85:1–4.
2. Hughes CA, Harley EH, Milmore G, Bala R, Martorella A. Birth trauma in the head and neck. Arch Otolaryngol Head Neck Surg 1999;125:193–9.

3. Evans AK, Licameli G, Brietzke S, Wittemore K, Kenna M. Pediatric facial nerve paralysis: patients, management and outcomes. Int J Pediatr Otorhinolaryngol 2005;69:1521–8.
4. Seddon HJ. A classification of nerve injuries. Br Med J 1942;2:237–9.
5. Sunderland S. A classification of peripheral nerve injury producing loss of function. Brain 1951;74:491–516.
6. Sunderland S, Cossar DF. The structure of the facial nerve. Anat Rec 1953;116:147–65.
7. May M, Fria RJ, Blumenthal F, Curtin H. Facial paralysis in children differential diagnosis. Otolaryngol Head Neck Surg 1981;89:841–8.
8. Lustig LR, Niparko JK. Disorders of the facial nerve. In: Lalwani AK, editor. Current Diagnosis & Treatment: Otolaryngology Head and Neck Surgery. New York: McGraw Hill Medical, 2008. pp. 847–72.
9. Renault F. Facial electromyography in newborn and young infants with congenital facial weakness. Dev Med Child Neurol 2001;43:421.
10. Sapin SO, Miller AA, Bass HN. Neonatal asymmetric crying facies: a new look at an old problem. Clin Pediatr 2005;44:109.

23 Bell's Palsy

A 37-year-old female presents for evaluation of sudden-onset left facial paralysis. She states that she had a cold last week with associated upper respiratory tract infection symptoms, malaise, and fatigue. She denies any associated otalgia, hearing loss, or vertigo. The day before while walking her dog in the evening, she reports having had some difficulty in calling her dog by whistling. She also noted abnormal discomfort in association with the sound of her dog barking. On awakening she noted complete left-sided facial paralysis and presented immediately for evaluation. She denies any previous episodes of facial paresis or paralysis. She reports difficulty in oral competency while consuming breakfast. She denies any additional neurologic symptoms including upper or lower extremity weakness, paresthesias, or changes in facial sensation. Past medical history is significant for exercise-induced asthma. There is no past trauma history. Her past surgical history is significant only for cholecystectomy 2 years prior. Medications include oral contraceptive and an albuterol inhaler. As for social history, she does not consume tobacco, alcohol, or recreational drug products. On physical examination, the patient is a thin 37-year-old female who appears her stated age. She is noted to have complete facial paralysis with no motion on attempt at eyebrow raise, eye closure with effort, snarl (wrinkling the nose), pursing lips, frown, and smile. The remainder of the head and neck examination including otoscopy was within normal limits.

What do you do now?

Idiopathic facial paresis, or Bell's palsy as it is more frequently called, is the most common cause of unilateral facial paralysis.[1] It is characterized by an acute onset of facial paresis or paralysis evolving over 24–48 hours associated with edema of the peripheral facial nerve leading to neuropraxia (conduction blockage) of the facial nerve of unknown etiology.[2-5] The presumed pathophysiology associated with Bell's palsy is one of inflammation and viral infection involving the facial nerve with subsequent edema of the facial nerve cause by either activation of a latent herpetic or varicella infection or a newly acquired upper respiratory tract virus.[5-10]

The annual incidence of Bell's palsy within the United States is approximately 11–40 cases per 100,000 population.[2,3,5,11,12] Similarly, the associated lifetime risk of Bell's palsy is approximately 1 in 60.[13] The clinical presentation of Bell's palsy may range from mild paresis to complete paralysis typically of acute unilateral onset involving all branches of the peripheral facial nerve leading to[14-16]

- Difficulty with eyebrow raise
- Difficulty with eye closure
- Difficulty making facial expressions
- Difficulty grimacing or smiling
- Oral incompetence or drooling
- Facial twitching

Patients often present with associated symptoms of[14-16]

- Otalgia (ear pain)
- Eye complaints including ophthalmalgia (eye pain), xerophthalmia (dry eye), or epiphora (abnormal tearing)
- Hyperacusis (discomfort with loud sounds)
- Dysgeusia (taste disturbance)
- Xerostomia (dry mouth)
- Headache

The diagnosis of Bell's palsy is made largely based on history and physical examination. Time course of onset of symptoms and lack of associated physical findings with the exception of facial paresis or paralysis in all branches guide the diagnosis. Although originally developed to grade outcomes in facial function following acoustic neuroma resection, the House-Brackmann grading scale has become widely used for the purpose of documenting presentation and outcomes in facial paralysis in association with Bell's palsy. Table 23-1 details the components of the House-Brachmann grading scale.[17] However, because Bell's palsy is a diagnosis of exclusion, one must have a keen awareness of the differential diagnosis associated with acute unilateral facial paralysis and screen for possible alternative etiologies either through history, physical examination, or additional testing modalities. Bell's palsy is differentiated from other causes of acute facial paralysis by its rapid progression and typical self-limiting course.[5] Additional disease processes to be considered within the differential diagnosis are presented in Table 23-2.

Additional testing for these disease entities should be guided by a high index of suspicion based on positive risk factors for disease (i.e., history of camping or deer hunting and Lyme disease, history of intravenous drug use or multiple transfusions and HIV infection, history of multiple unprotected sexual partners and syphilis), key symptoms noted on history (i.e., unilateral hearing loss from skull base tumors, facial swelling from parotid tumors), and consistent physical findings on examination (i.e., nasal crusting and perforation from Wegener's granulomatosis, suppurative middle ear effusion from acute otitis media, vesicular rash from Ramsay Hunt syndrome). Although not compulsory in the diagnostic evaluation of isolated episode of Bell's palsy, magnetic resonance imaging if obtained may reveal enhancement of the facial nerve with gadolinium staining. Magnetic resonance imaging is, however, recommended for cases of recurrent Bell's palsy, Bell's palsy with unsatisfactory facial outcome, bilateral Bell's palsy, or if the clinical index of suspicion is high for an alternative pathology as the etiologic factor for facial paralysis.

The natural history of Bell's palsy is one of self-limited edema of the facial nerve with spontaneous resolution of facial palsy completely in approximately 70% of cases and to near-normal function in approximately 85% of cases.[14-16] As such, 20%–30% of individuals maintain some degree of less than desirable facial function, which may be associated with psychological or emotional stress and trauma. Age greater than 60 years and previous diagnosis of diabetes mellitus have been associated with a poorer prognosis for facial function.[14-16]

All patients presenting with Bell's palsy should be instructed regarding the importance of eye care. Patients should be urged to use artificial

TABLE 23-1 **House-Brackmann Facial Nerve Grading System**[17]

Grade	Description	Eye Closure	Forehead Movement	Mouth Movement	Synkinesis	Symmetry at Rest	Gross Movement
1	Normal	Yes	Normal	Normal	No	Yes	Normal
2	Mild dysfunction	Yes	Moderate to good	Slight asymmetry	Very slight	Yes	Slight weakness noticeable on close inspection
3	Moderate dysfunction	Yes with effort	Slight to moderate	Slight weakness with maximum effort	Yes	Yes	Obvious weakness, not disfiguring
4	Moderate-severe dysfunction	No	None	Asymmetric with maximum effort	Yes	Yes	Obvious weakness and/or disfiguring asymmetry
5	Severe dysfunction	No	None	Slight	Yes	No	Barely perceivable
6	Total paralysis	No	None	None	N/A	No	None

N/A, not applicable.

TABLE 23-2 **Differential Diagnosis of Unilateral Facial Paralysis**

Differential Diagnosis of Unilateral Facial Paralysis

Otologic	Systemic
Acute mastoiditis	Sarcoidosis
Acute otitis media	Diabetes mellitus
Cholesteatoma	Amyloidosis
Malignant otitis externa	Guillain-Barré syndrome
Skull base osteomyelitis	Melkersson-Rosenthal syndrome
	Wegener's granulomatosis
Central nervous system	Neoplastic
Pontine lesion	Facial nerve schwannoma
Cerebrovascular accident	Vestibular schwannoma
Vertebral artery aneurysm	Glomus tumor
Basilar artery aneurysm	Lymphoma
	Parotid gland tumor
Infectious	Meningioma
Lyme disease	
HIV infection	Trauma
Syphilis	Temporal bone fracture

tear drops regularly, to place ophthalmologic moisturizing ointment in the affected eye at night, and to use protective eyewear (i.e., goggles when outdoors because they are unable to protect their eye from debris in the wind). Taping of the eye should be done with great care to ensure that the eyelashes do not become trapped adjacent to the cornea increasing the risk of corneal abrasion. Improper eye care may lead to corneal injury, ophthalmologic infection, and ultimately blindness in the affected eye. If there is a concern for corneal abrasion or improper eye care, ophthalmology consultation should be obtained.

Because of the association between facial nerve edema and potential viral etiology, systemic corticosteroid and antiviral therapy remains the mainstay of treatment for Bell's palsy. A 5- to 10-day course of high-dose antiviral therapy (i.e., acyclovir, 2,000–2,400 mg daily; famciclovir, 250 mg daily; or valacyclovir, 1,000–3,000 mg daily) is typically used with an average dose of 1 mg/kg/day of prednisone or its equivalent for 7–10 days followed by a taper.[18-24]

In a meta-analysis of 18 clinical trials comprised of a total of 2,786 patients, the efficacy of steroids alone, antivirals alone, and combination therapy compared with placebo were assessed.[25] Corticosteroids alone were associated with a risk reduction in unsatisfactory recovery (relative risk, 0.69; 95% confidence interval, 0.55–0.87; $P = 0.001$), reduction in risk of synkinesis and autonomic dysfunction (relative risk, 0.48; 95% confidence interval, 0.36–0.65; $P < 0.001$) with no increase in adverse effects. The associated number needed to treat to benefit was 11. Antiviral agents alone were not associated with a reduction in risk of unsatisfactory recovery ($P = 0.48$). However, in combination, corticosteroids and antiviral agents were associated with a greater risk reduction than corticosteroids alone (relative risk, 0.75; 95% confidence interval, 0.56–1.00; $P = 0.05$).

More commonly performed in previous decades, surgical decompression of the facial nerve in association with Bell's palsy has become somewhat controversial. The results of electroneuronography, which assesses for asymmetry in facial function and the presence of wallerian degeneration, and voluntary electromyography are most critical in surgical decision making. Evidence of greater than 90% degeneration on electroneuronography testing and no voluntary motor unit electromyography potentials within 14 days of onset are the surgical criteria most commonly used.[26] Decompression in this population has been associated with 91% House-Brackmann grade I or II outcomes. However, a recent Cochrane Database review of facial nerve decompression in Bell's palsy revealed insufficient evidence to support or refute its use in the treatment of patients with Bell's palsy.[27] As such, because recovery rates remain good without surgical intervention, decompression is commonly reserved for patients with recurrent paralysis, history of contralateral facial dysfunction, or other special circumstances.[5]

There currently are no established preventive therapies for Bell's palsy. Recovery from Bell's palsy typically occurs within the first 2 weeks to 6 months following the onset of symptoms. During the days or weeks of symptomatology, eye protection is key.

> **KEY POINTS TO REMEMBER**
> - Bell's palsy is idiopathic facial paresis.
> - Bell's palsy is the most common cause of unilateral facial paralysis.
> - Patients should be screened by history and physical examination and directed studies for alternative etiologies of facial paralysis.
> - Complete resolution of palsy occurs in 70% of patients, with near complete resolution in 85% of patients.
> - The mainstay of treatment includes oral steroids and antivirals.

Further Reading
1. Gilden DH. Bell's palsy: clinical practice. N Engl J Med 2004;351:1323–31.
2. Gronseth GS, Paduga R. Evidence-based guideline update: steroids and antivirals for Bell palsy. Report of the Guideline Development Subcommittee of the American Academy of Neurology. Neurology 2012;79:2209–13.
3. Hauser WA, Karnes WE, Annis J, Kurland LT. Incidence and prognosis of Bell's palsy in the population of Rochester, Minnesota. Mayo Clin Proc 1971;46:258–64.
4. Cawthorne T. The pathology and surgical treatment of Bell's palsy. Proc R Soc Med 1950;4:565–72.
5. Danner CJ. Facial nerve paralysis. Otolaryngol Clin N Am 2008;41:619–32.
6. Adour KK, Bell DN, Hilsinger RL Jr. Herpes simplex virus in idiopathic facial paralysis (Bell palsy). JAMA 1975;233:527–30.
7. Stjernquist-Desatnik A, Skoog E, Aurelius E. Detection of herpes simplex and varicella zoster viruses in patients with Bell's palsy by polymerase chain reaction techniques. Ann Otol Rhinol Laryngol 2006;115:306–11.
8. Theil D, Arbusow V, Derfuss R, et al. Prevalence of HSV-1 LAT in human trigeminal, geniculate and vestibular ganglia and its implication for cranial nerve syndromes. Brain Pathol 2001;11:408–13.
9. Furuta Y, Fukuda S, Suzuki S, et al. Detection of varicella-zoster virus DNA in patients with acute peripheral facial palsy by the polymerase chain reaction and its use for early diagnosis of zoster sine herpete. J Med Virol 1997;52:316–9.
10. Hato N, Murakami S, Gyo K. Steroid and antiviral treatment of Bell's palsy. Lancet 2008;371:1818–20.

11. DeDiego-Sastre JI, Prim-Espada MP, Fernandez-Garcia F. The epidemiology of Bell's palsy. Rev Neurol 2005;41:287–90.
12. Quant EC, Jeste SS, Muni RH, et al. The benefits of steroids versus steroids plus antivirals for treatment of Bell's palsy: a meta-analysis. BMJ 2009;339:b3354–60.
13. Holland NJ, Weiner GM. Recent developments in Bell's palsy. BMJ 2004;329:553–7.
14. Adour KK, Wingerd J. Idiopathic facial paralysis (Bell's palsy): factors affecting severity and outcome in 446 patients. Neurology 1974;24:112–6.
15. Peitersen E. The natural history of Bell's palsy. Am J Otol 1982;4:107–11.
16. Devriese PP, Schumacher T, Scheide A, DeJongh RH, Houtkooper JM. Incidence, prognosis and recovery of Bell's palsy. Clin Otolaryngol 1990;15:15–7.
17. House JW, Brackmann DE. Facial nerve grading system. Otolaryngol Head Neck Surg 1985;93:146–7.
18. Adour KK, Ruboyianes JM, Von Doersten PG, et al. Bell's palsy treatment with acyclovir and prednisone compared with prednisone alone: a double-blind, randomized, controlled trial. Ann Otol Rhinol Laryngol 1996;105:371–8.
19. Hato N, Yamada H, Kohno H, et al. Valacyclovir and prednisolone treatment for Bell's palsy: a multicenter, randomized, placebo-controlled study. Otol Neurotol 2007;28:408–13.
20. Sullivan FM, Swan IR, Donnan PT, et al. Early treatment with prednisolone and acyclovir in Bell's palsy. N Engl J Med 2007;357:1598–607.
21. Engstrom M, Berg T, Stjemquist-Desatnik A, et al. Prednisolone and valacyclovir in Bell's palsy: a randomized, double-blind, placebo-controlled, multicenter trial. Lancet Neurol 2008;7:993–1000.
22. Kawaguchi K, Inamura H, Abe Y, et al. Reactivation of herpes simplex type 1 and varicella-zoster virus and therapeutic effects of combination therapy with prednisolone and valacyclovir in patients in Bell's palsy. Laryngoscope 2007;117:147-56.
23. Minnerop M, Herbst M, Fimmers R, et al. Bell's palsy: combined treatment of famciclovir and prednisone is superior to prednisone alone. J Neurol 2008;255:1726–30.
24. Yeo SG, Lee YC, Park DC, Cha CI. Acyclovir plus steroid versus steroid alone in the treatment of Bell's palsy. Am J Otolaryngol 2008;29:163–6.
25. de Almeida JR, Al Khabori M, Guyatt GH, et al. Combination corticosteroid and antiviral treatment for Bell Palsy: a systematic review and meta-analysis. JAMA 2009;302:985–93.
26. Gantz BJ, Rubinstein JT, Gidley P, Woodworth GG. Surgical management of Bell's palsy. Laryngoscope 1999;109:1177–88.
27. McAllister K, Walker D, Donnan PT, Swan I. Surgical interventions for the early management of Bell's palsy. Cochrane Database Syst Rev. 2011;16:CD007468.

24 Traumatic Facial Palsy

A 42-year-old male was brought in by ambulance to the local trauma hospital following penetrating trauma to the left temporal bone. The patient was stabbed with a butcher knife in the left temporal region by a friend during an argument. On evaluation by the emergency medical team, the patient was noted to be obtunded. He was immediately intubated in the field. Facial nerve function was not documented. The patient on arrival at the local trauma hospital underwent computed tomography of the head, which revealed an intracranial hemorrhage and penetration of the temporal bone. This revealed a tract of penetration from the knife, which terminates in the region of the geniculate ganglion. On awakening and extubation, the patient was noted to have complete left facial paralysis. He also revealed complaints of decreased hearing on the left. Past medical history was significant for hypertension. There is no past surgical or trauma history. Medications include a diuretic for management of hypertension. As for social history, he consumes 20–30 alcoholic beverages per week and has smoked one pack per day of cigarettes for the past 20 years. He denies recreational drug use. Physical examination revealed House-Brackmann 6 facial function on the left and House-Brackmann 1 facial function on the right. The physical examination was also significant for a Weber that lateralized to the left and Rinne that has bone better than air (negative) sound conduction on the left. Dedicated computed tomography of the temporal bone is presented in Figure 24-1.

What do you do now?

Facial nerve injury is a potential complication of temporal bone fractures associated with temporal bone trauma. Temporal bone trauma may be classified as either blunt or penetrating. Most temporal bone fractures secondary to temporal bone trauma occur as a function of blunt trauma.

PENETRATING TEMPORAL BONE TRAUMA

Penetrating trauma accounts for only a small proportion of temporal bone trauma. In most series, penetrating trauma accounts for less that 10% of temporal bone trauma; however, rates as high as 30% have been reported.[1-7] Most commonly, penetrating temporal bone trauma takes the form of gunshots as the mechanism of trauma. Facial nerve palsy has been associated with 36%–50% of surviving patients following penetrating temporal bone trauma.[8-10] The most common location of facial nerve transection following penetrating temporal bone trauma is within the tympanic (middle ear or horizontal) and mastoid (descending) segment of the facial nerve. In most cases, facial palsy presents immediately

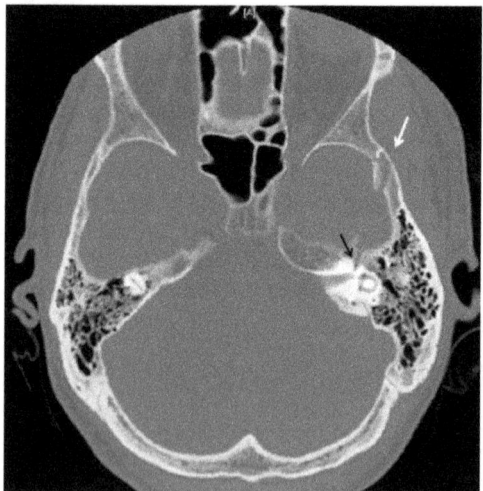

FIGURE 24-1 Penetrating temporal bone injury. Axial computed tomography scan of temporal bones without contrast on bone windows demonstrating penetrating trauma to the temporal bone with involvement of the facial nerve. The *white arrow* highlights the injury caused by the entry point of the knife; the *black arrow* depicts violation of the facial nerve at the genu.

and represents transection of the facial nerve. However, these patients are commonly afflicted with significant comorbid injury resulting in a comatose state. In such cases electrophysiologic testing of nerve integrity may be performed to confirm facial nerve transection.[10] Operative repair of transected nerve should be performed as soon as the patient is deemed medically stable, as was performed in the patient described in the case in this chapter. Operative repair may include anastomosis, sectioning of nonviable nerve tissue, and cable grafting (interposing a free graft of neural tissue obtained from an autologous donor site, such as the greater auricular or sural nerves). Concomitant hearing loss may be addressed with amplification or reconstruction of the eardrum and ossicular chain.

BLUNT TEMPORAL BONE TRAUMA

Temporal bone fractures occurring secondary to blunt temporal bone trauma are typically classified according to one of two classification systems: by axis of the temporal bone involved or by otic capsule involvement. The former represents the traditional classification system proposed by Ulrich in 1926.[11] The later represents a more contemporary classification system that has been noted to have a higher prognostic significance.

According to the traditional classification system proposed by Ulrich, temporal bone fractures are categorized as longitudinal or transverse.[11,12] Longitudinal fractures parallel the long axis of the petrous pyramid and are associated with a temporoparietal vector of trauma force (Figure 24-2). Longitudinal fractures using this classification system have been reported to be associated with approximately 80% of temporal bone fractures.[1,5-6,12,13] Among longitudinal temporal bone fractures, facial nerve injury has been reported in approximately 10%–25% of fractures.[7,13,14] Transverse fractures are oriented perpendicular to the long axis of the petrous pyramid (Figure 24-3) and are associated with a fronto-occipital vector of trauma force. Transverse fractures using this classification system have been reported to be associated with approximately 20% of temporal bone fractures.[1,5,6,12,13] Among transverse temporal bone fractures, facial nerve injury has been reported in approximately 35%–50% of fractures.[7,13,14]

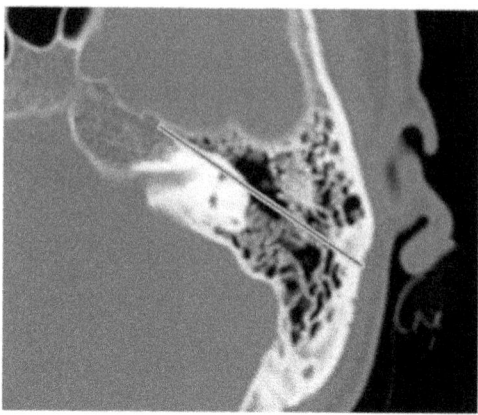

FIGURE 24-2 Longitudinal temporal bone fracture. Axial computed tomography scan of temporal bones without contrast on bone windows demonstrating the orientation of a longitudinal temporal bone fracture (*grey line*) involving the geniculate ganglion.

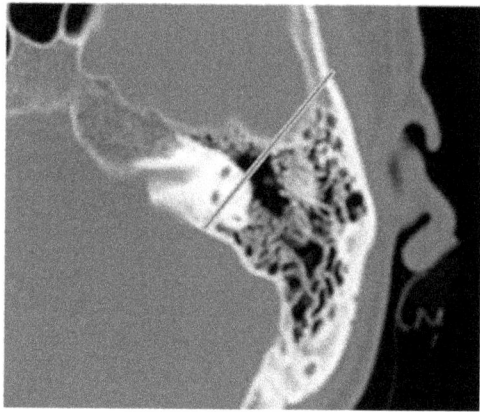

FIGURE 24-3 Transverse temporal bone fracture. Axial computed tomography scan of temporal bones without contrast on bone windows demonstrating the orientation of a transverse temporal bone fracture (*grey line*).

However, all temporal bone fractures do not strictly adhere to this classification system. For this reason modifications to the axis classification system were developed including oblique (Figure 24-4) and mixed temporal bone fractures, which in certain series account for a large proportion of temporal bone fractures.[2,3,15]

An alternative classification system for temporal bone fractures has gained popularity because it has been noted to be of increased diagnostic and clinical significance. This system classifies temporal bone fractures according to their relation to the otic capsule. The otic capsule is the dense bony encasement of inner ear (Figure 24-5). Within this classification system, temporal bones are classified as otic capsule violating (Figure 24-6) or otic capsule sparing (Figure 24-7). Using this classification system in most series, otic capsule–sparing fractures have been found to comprise greater than 90% of temporal bone fractures.[3,4,16] Otic capsule–violating temporal

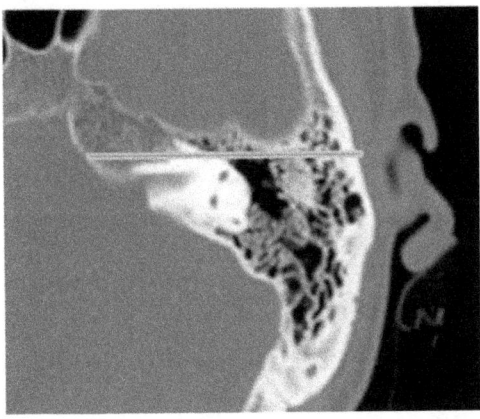

FIGURE 24-4 Oblique temporal bone fracture. Axial computed tomography scan of temporal bones without contrast on bone windows demonstrating the orientation of an oblique temporal bone fracture (*grey line*).

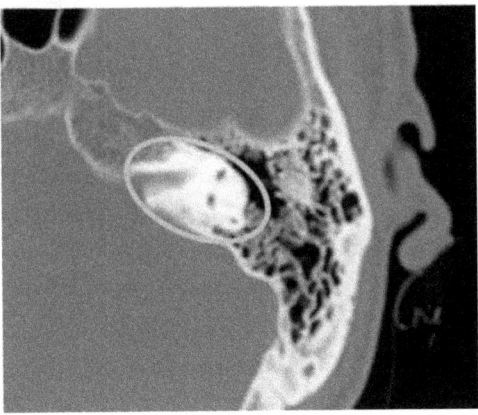

FIGURE 24-5 Otic capsule. Axial computed tomography scan of temporal bones without contrast on bone windows. The *grey circle* highlights the structures comprising the otic capsule of the temporal bone.

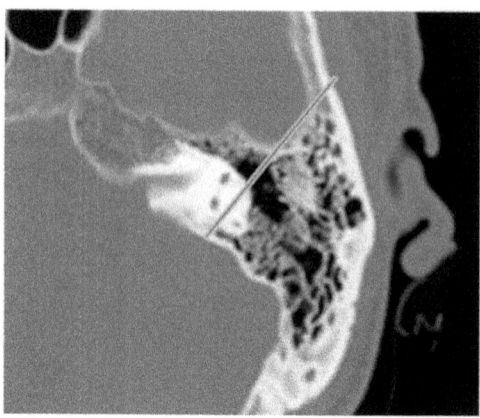

FIGURE 24-6 Otic capsule–violating temporal bone fracture.

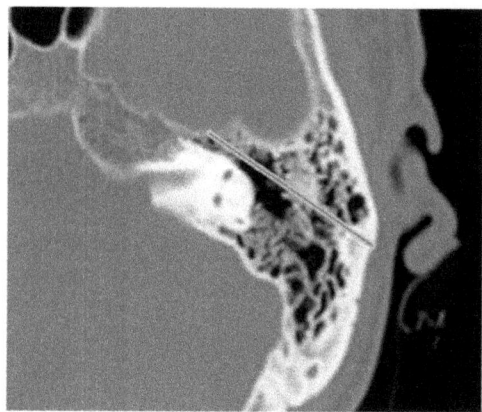

FIGURE 24-7 Otic capsule–sparing temporal bone fracture.

bone fractures are associated with a two to five times greater risk of facial nerve injury versus the less than 10% of otic capsule–sparing temporal bone fractures being associated with facial nerve involvement.[3,4,7] Trauma involving the otic capsule invariably leads to profound sensorineural hearing loss. Other trauma may disrupt the ossicular chain, tympanic membrane, and external ear canal resulting in hemotypanum and conductive hearing deficits.

The most important factor in evaluating patients following temporal bone trauma and possible facial nerve injury is immediate documentation of facial function. This has the most significant impact on clinical management. Immediate facial palsy may be defined as facial palsy noted immediately following the trauma event. This is highly suggestive of facial nerve transection or impingement. Delayed facial palsy may be defined as facial palsy that develops progressively hours to days following the traumatic event and is believed to represent edema of the nerve. In a review by Brodie and Thompson[4] of patients with facial palsy following temporal bone trauma, more than 70% of patients presented with delayed facial paralysis. However, in a significant proportion of patients, immediate facial nerve function cannot be documented. Often, these patients have many other life-threatening injuries that take priority in their care or the individuals are comatose precluding examination of facial function.[10]

The most common location of injury following blunt temporal bone trauma is at the geniculate ganglion followed by second genu. However, injury can occur at any location within the temporal bone. Partial or incomplete facial palsy may represent edema of the nerve, concussion, hematoma, impingement by bony fragments, or partial nerve transection.

The management of delayed facial nerve palsy is controversial. For delayed facial paralysis in both blunt and penetrating temporal bone trauma, most neurotologists recommend conservative management including watchful waiting and high-dose corticosteroids. Similarly, patients with partial facial palsy are managed conservatively.

Electrophysiologic studies are of benefit in assessing patients with immediate facial palsy following blunt temporal bone trauma. There is controversy regarding the use of electrophysiologic studies in patients with delayed complete facial palsy; however, this is advocated by some specialists. Elecrophysiologic testing is performed 72 hours following injury to allow time for nerve fibers distal to the site of injury to degenerate. The most commonly used eletrophysiologic studies are

- Electroneuronography (ENOG): This test assesses evoked myogenic potential in the muscles of facial expression following stimulation of the facial nerves bilaterally. The difference in the amplitude of myogenic potential is reported.

- Nerve excitability test: Nerve stimulator probes are placed at the stylomastoid foramen. The current is slowly increased until facial twitch is just visible. A difference of 3.5 mA between sides indicates a loss of greater than 90% neural integrity.
- Voluntary electromyography: This test requires the patient to be awake and able to follow commands. This test assesses evoked myogenic potential in the muscles of facial expression with voluntary attempts at facial motion. The presence of fibrillation potentials indicates axonal degenerations, but do not appear until 10–14 days postinjury.

Surgical intervention is not indicated in patients with[17]

- Documented normal facial nerve function after injury regardless of progression
- Presentation of incomplete facial paralysis with no progression to complete paralysis
- Degeneration of less than 95% on ENOG studies

In blunt trauma, facial nerve decompression may be used when ENOG criteria reveal a significant degree of wallerian degeneration. In a study of 66 patients who underwent facial nerve decompression secondary to temporal bone trauma, 47% of patients achieved House-Brackmann grade 1 facial nerve function with 92.9% of patients achieving House-Brackmann 1 or 2 facial outcome when decompression was performed within the first 2 weeks of injury.[18] These outcomes were found to be statistically significantly better than patients who received decompression at greater than 2 weeks ($P < .01$).[18] Late decompression surgery is not typically recommended.[17] As such in current practice within the United States, facial nerve decompression is infrequently performed. Given the nature of disease in trauma patients and associated comorbidities, immediate documentation of facial function is often challenging. Additionally documentation of facial injury on recovery of associated intracranial injury often falls outside of the window of decompression. When transection of the nerve is encountered and operative repair of the nerve is required, long-term recovery with a moderate deficit and complete eye closure or better is obtained in approximately 80% of patients on repair.[19,20]

CASE CONTINUED

ENOG was performed at 10 days postinjury and the patient was noted to have 97% degeneration. Operative management was used via the middle fossa approach and the patient was noted to have transection of the facial nerve at the genu, which was repaired by neural grafting techniques (cable graft using the greater auricular nerve).

Permanent sensorineural hearing loss post temporal bone fracture is addressed with amplification. Conductive hearing loss may also be habituated with amplification; however, most patients opt for surgery, which is highly successful in repairing torn eardrums and the reconstruction of the ossicular chain.

KEY POINTS TO REMEMBER

- Traumatic facial palsy may occur in association with temporal bone fractures
- The most common location of facial nerve transection following penetrating temporal bone trauma is within the tympanic (middle ear or horizontal) and mastoid (descending) segment of the facial nerve
- Facial paralysis is more commonly associated with transverse temporal bone fractures
- Facial nerve status should be documented as soon as possible when treating patients with temporal bone trauma
- Steroids should be given early in the course

Further Reading

1. Cannon CR, Jahrsdoerfer RA. Temporal bone fractures. Review of 90 cases. Arch Otolaryngol 1983;109:285–8.
2. Alvi A, Bereliani A. Acute intracranial complications of temporal bone trauma. Otolaryngol Head Neck Surg 1998;119:609–13.
3. Dahiya R, Keller JD, Litofsky NS, et al. Temporal bone fractures: otic capsule sparing versus otic capsule violating clinical and radiographic considerations. J Trauma 1999;47:1079–83.
4. Brodie HA, Thompson TC. Management of complications for 820 temporal bone fractures. Am J Otol 1997;18:188–97.

5. Ishman SL, Friedland DR. Temporal bone fractures: traditional classification and clinical relevance. Laryngoscope 2004;114:1734–41.
6. Lee D, Honrado C, Har-El G, et al. Pediatric temporal bone fractures. Laryngoscope 1998;108:816–21.
7. Little SC, Kesser BW. Radiographic classification of temporal bone fractures: clinical predictability using a new system. Arch Otolaryngol Head Neck Surg 2006;132:1300–4.
8. Bento RF, de Brito RV. Gunshot wounds to the facial nerve. Otol Neurotol 2004;25:1009–13.
9. Backous DD, Minor LB, Niparko JK. Trauma to the external auditory canal and temporal bone. Otolaryngol Clin North Am 1996;29:853–66.
10. Oghalai JS. Temporal bone trauma. In: Lalwani AK, editor. Current Diagnosis & Treatment: Otolaryngology Head and Neck Surgery. New York: McGraw Hill Medical, 2008. pp. 744–52.
11. Ulrich K. Verletzungen des gohororgans bei schadelbasisfrakturen (eine histologische und klinisshe studie). Acta Otolaryngol Suppl 1926;6:1–150.
12. Gurdjian ES, Webster JE. Deformation of the skull in head injury studies by stresscoat technique. Surg Gynecol Obstet 1946;83:219–33.
13. Johnson F, Semaan MT, Megerian CA. Temporal bone fracture: evaluation and management in the modern era. Otolaryngol Clin N Am 2008;41:597–618.
14. Nosan DK, Benecke JE Jr, Murr AH. Current perspective on temporal bone trauma. Otolaryngol Head Neck Surg 1997;117:67–71.
15. Ghorayeb BY, Yeakley JW, Hall JW III, et al. Unusual complications of temporal bone fractures. Arch Otolaryngol Head Neck Surg 1987;113:749–53.
16. Rafferty MA, McConn-Walsh R, Walsh MA. A comparison of temporal bone fracture classification systems. Clin Otolaryngol 2006;31:287–91.
17. Chang CY, Cass SP. Management of facial nerve injury due to temporal bone trauma. Am J Otol 1999;20:96–114.
18. Hato N, Nota J, Hakuba N, Gyo K, Yanaqihara N. Facial nerve decompression surgery in patients with temporal bone trauma. J Trauma 2011;71:1789–92.
19. Darrouzet V, Duclas JY, Liguoro D, et al. Management of facial paralysis resulting from temporal bone fractures: our experience in 115 cases. Otolaryngol Head Neck Surg 2001;125:77–84.
20. Ulug T, Arif Ulubil S. Management of facial paralysis in temporal bone fractures: a prospective study analyzing 11 operated fractures. Am J Otolaryngol 2005;26:230–8.

25 Facial Neuroma

A 47-year-old female presented for evaluation of "recurrent Bell's palsy." The patient stated that she has had two episodes of left-sided Bell's palsy over the course of the past 5 years. She denied previous history of magnetic resonance imaging (MRI) scan or laboratory investigation in association with episodes. She stated that she was previously treated with corticosteroids and antiviral medications with near complete return of function with only mild synkinesis. She presented in consultation for evaluation of left facial paralysis not resolving within 8 weeks following treatment with corticosteroids and antiviral medications. She reported progressive decline in hearing on the left side over the course of the past year with inability to use the telephone on the left. She has mild high-frequency, nonpulsatile fluctuating tinnitus. Past medical history was significant for seasonal allergies. There was no past surgical or trauma history. Medications included oral contraceptive and an antihistamine. As for social history, she did not use tobacco. She consumed one to two glasses of red wine weekly. She denied recreational drug use. She consumed six to seven cups of caffeinated beverages daily including coffee and soda. Her daily sodium consumption was greater than 4,000 mg/day, and she consumed less than one glass of water per day. Physical examination revealed complete left-sided facial paralysis (House-Brackmann 6) with normal facial function on the right (House-Brackmann 1). The remainder of the physical examination was unremarkable. Pure tone audiogram is presented in Figure 25-1. Her speech discrimination score was 40% on the left and 100% on the right. MRI of the internal auditory canals was obtained, revealing a lesion filling the lateral internal auditory canal, which was isointense on T1-weighted imaging, hypointense on T2-weighted imaging (Figure 25-2), and enhanced with gadolinium contrast.

What do you do now?

Neuromas of the facial nerve are rare tumors involving the temporal bone. The prevalence of facial neuroma is believed to be approximately 0.15%–0.8%.[1-4] Most facial neuromas are derived from Schwann cell origin and are thus also commonly known as facial schwannomas.

Facial schwannomas are extremely slow-growing tumors with a slight male preponderance typically presenting during middle age.[4,5] The most common sites of involvement for facial schwannoma include the geniculate region, labyrinthine segment, and tympanic segment of the facial nerve within most series.[6-8] However, facial schwannoma can develop anywhere along the course of the facial nerve.[4,9] In fact, facial schwannoma commonly involves more than one segment of the facial nerve.[4,10]

The clinical presentation of patients with facial schwannoma can vary greatly. Because of the overlapping clinical manifestation between facial schwannoma and vestibular schwannoma, and the relatively rare occurrence of facial schwannoma, misdiagnosis as vestibular schwannoma may occur. The most common symptom of facial schwannoma is facial palsy.[2,4]

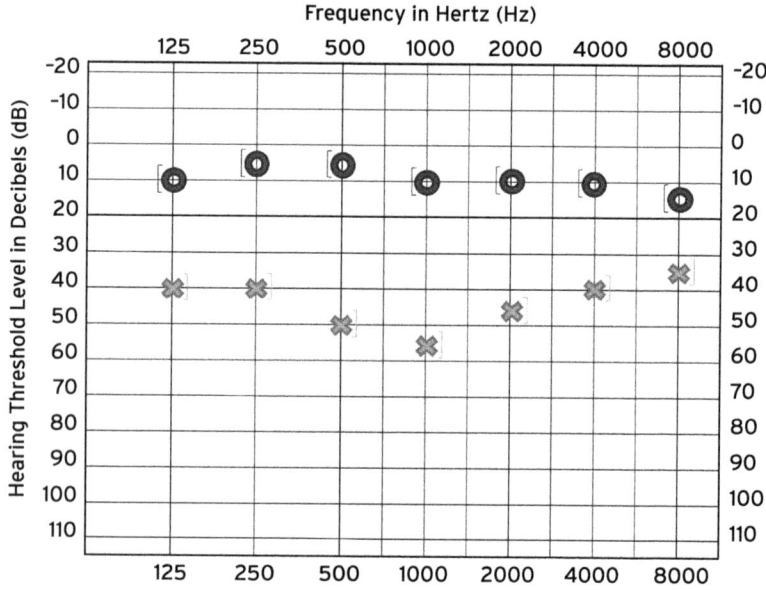

FIGURE 25-1 Pure tone audiogram from patient with recurrent facial paralysis indicates a moderately severe left asymmetric sensorineural hearing loss.

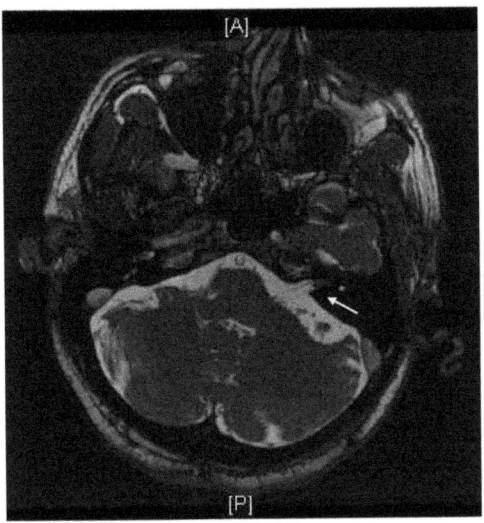

FIGURE 25-2 Axial T2-weighted MRI scan from patient with recurrent left facial paralysis. The *white arrow* highlights a lesion filling the lateral left internal auditory canal.

However, patients with facial schwannoma may present with any of the following symptoms:

- Asymptomatic incidental finding on imaging
- Facial paresis or paralysis (often recurrent)
- Hearing loss (conductive, mixed, or sensorineural)
- Tinnitus
- Hemifacial spasm
- Dysgeusia
- Hyperacusis

Similarly, on physical examination, findings may vary in patients with facial schwannoma. However, the most common clinical findings on examination are facial paresis, facial paralysis, and hemifacial spasm. Patients may present with hearing loss as manifested by abnormalities on tuning fork examination. In cases of tympanic segment involvement, middle ear mass may be present on otoscopy. Typically, the remainder of the physical examination is unremarkable.

The differential diagnosis for facial schwannoma includes any mass lesion of the internal auditory canal, mastoid, or middle ear. However, the following lesions may present with symptomatology and radiographic findings resembling that of facial schwannoma:

- Vestibular schwannoma (acoustic neuroma)
- Facial hemangioma
- Meningioma
- Metastasis from primary breast, kidney, lung, or stomach malignancies
- Lesion from perineural invasion of local squamous cell carcinoma or parotid mucoepidermoid carcinoma
- Paragangliomas (i.e., glomus tympanicum)
- Cholesterol granuloma
- Epidermoid cyst

The diagnostic evaluation of patients with suspected facial schwannoma should include a thin-cut MRI of the temporal bones and posterior fossa. MRI is of assistance in differentiating facial schwannoma from most other tumors included within the differential.[4,6,8] The imaging characteristics of facial schwannoma on MRI are similar to that of vestibular schwannoma making it challenging to differentiate for clinicians without specialization and expertise in neuroradiology. Typically, facial schwannoma presents as isointense or hypointense on T1-weighted imaging. Similarly, T2-weighted imaging reveals an isointense or hypointense lesion. These lesions avidly enhance with gadolinium contrast. Assisting in the diagnosis of facial schwannoma is the course of the lesion, particularly given that a significant percentage of tumors have some involvement of the labyrinthine segment of the nerve, which is not characteristic of vestibular schwannoma. Additionally, high-resolution, thin-cut computed tomography imaging of the temporal bone can provide additional information to assist in the diagnosis. Computed tomography imaging of the temporal bone provides additional detail regarding the course of the facial nerve, widening of its bony canal, increased diameter of the nerve, tumor margins, and involvement or erosion of adjacent structures in patients with facial schwannoma (Figure 25-3). Additionally, audiometric evaluation including pure tone audiometry, speech discrimination scores, and stapedial reflexes should be obtained. Facial nerve electrophysiologic studies can be of assistance in identifying facial nerve involvement, but are not routinely obtained.

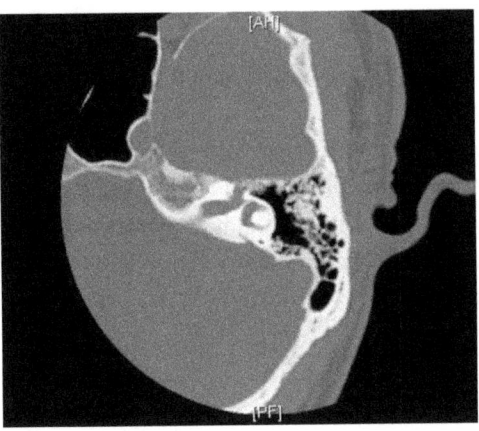

FIGURE 25-3 Axial CT scan of the left temporal bone on bone windows from patient with recurrent facial paralysis. The *white* highlights widening of the fallopian canal of the facial nerve indicating mass effect of a lesion likely involving the facial nerve.

The treatment of facial schwannoma is somewhat controversial in terms of timing and modality of therapy. Typically, in asymptomatic patients with small tumors, observation alone is recommended with serial MRI scans and close follow-up.[2] Surgical resection is associated with the risk of facial palsy. Thus, some surgeons advocate for delayed operative management until moderate facial palsy from disease progression has transpired.[2,6] Alternatively, others advocate for early resection to preserve hearing and report superior results with facial reconstruction.[4,11] Following resection, facial nerve grafting is used for facial reanimation. Because of the rare nature of this tumor, there are not adequate data available to support early versus late operative management in facial schwannoma. For this reason, patients should be carefully counseled regarding the treatment options and allowed to participate in the decision process based on their personal preferences and beliefs. In larger tumors with significant associated morbidity and compression of vital structures, this dilemma is less pronounced. More recently, stereotactic radiosurgery has emerged as a potential alternative therapy in the treatment of facial nerve schwannoma.[12-14] Currently, available data reveal promise in stereotactic radiosurgery as a means of controlling tumor growth in facial schwannoma. However, long-term data regarding outcomes in stereotactic radiosurgery in the treatment of facial nerve schwannoma remain pending.

> **KEY POINTS TO REMEMBER**
>
> - Facial neuromas are rare tumors with a prevalence of approximately 0.15%–0.8%
> - Facial neuromas are slow-growing presenting asymptomatically or with hearing loss, tinnitus, facial spasm, dysgeusia, and hyperacusis
> - The treatment of facial schwannoma is controversial in terms of timing and modality of therapy and may include resection or stereotactic radiosurgery

Further Reading

1. Chung JW, Ahn JH, Kim JH, et al. Facial nerve schwannomas: different manifestations and outcomes. Surg Neurol 2004;62:245–52.
2. Falcioni M, Russo A, Taibah A, Sanna M. Facial nerve tumors. Otol Neurotol 2003;24:942–7.
3. Kida Y, Yoshimoto M, Hasegawa T. Radiosurgery for facial schwannoma. J Neurosurg 2007;106:24–9.
4. King TT, Morrison AW. Primary facial nerve tumors within the skull. J Neurosurg 1990;72:1–8.
5. Kubota Y, Kawamata T, Kubo O, et al. Large facial nerve schwannomas without facial palsy: case reports and review of the literature. Neurosurg Rev 2005;28:234–8.
6. Lipkin AF, Coker NJ, Jenkins HA, Alford BR. Intracranial and intratemporal facial neuroma. Otolaryngol Head Neck Surg 1987;96:71–9.
7. Litre CF, Gourg GP, Tamura M, et al. Gamma knife surgery for facial nerve schwannomas. Neurosurgery 2007;60:853–9.
8. Madhok R, Kondziolka D, Flickinger JC, Lunsford LD. Gamma knife radiosurgery for facial schwannomas. Neurosurgery 2009;64:1102–5.
9. McMonagle B, Al-Sanosi A, Croxson G, et al. Facial schwannoma: results of a large case series and review. J Laryngol Otol 2008;122:1139–50.
10. Perez R, Chen JM, Nedzelski JM. Intratemporal facial nerve schwannoma: a management dilemma. Otol Neurotol 2005;25:121–6.
11. Pulec JL. Symposium on ear surgery: facial nerve neuroma. Laryngoscope 1972;82:1160–76.
12. Saleh E, Achilli V, Naguib M, et al. Facial nerve neuromas: diagnosis and treatment. Am J Otol 1995;16:521–6.
13. Schmidt PH. Intratemporal neurinoma of the facial nerve. Pract Otorhinolaryngol (Basel) 1965;27:127–37.
14. Symon L, Cheesman AD, Kawauchi M, Bordt L. Neuromas of the facial nerve: a report of 12 cases. Br J Neurosurg 1993;7:13–22.

# SECTION V

Neurologic Complications of Otitis Media

26 Facial Paralysis

A 38-year-old man presents with acute onset of left facial weakness for several hours' duration. He has been on two antibiotics for otitis media. His facial function was nearly normal on awakening; however, within 3–4 hours his weakness has progressed to a House-Brackmann 6. The House-Brackmann grading system[1] for describing peripheral facial nerve (FN) weakness is the most universally used scale. In brief, and as seen in Table 26-1, grade 1 is normal function; 6 is complete lack of ipsilateral FN muscular function (all divisions); 2 is near normal function; 5 is nearly absent function with minimal presence of volitional movement; 3 is weakness at rest with closure of eye with maximal effort, and preserved (but weak) forehead movement; and 4 is weakness at rest, some eye closure with maximal effort, and absent forehead movement. Using the House-Brackmann scale enables for accurate description of progression or regression of weakness, and for accurate communication between healthcare providers. Examination reveals a healthy-appearing man with a House-Brackmann grade 6 left facial paralysis and left otitis media. There are no vesicles or eruptions seen around the pinna. Audiogram reveals moderate conductive hearing loss on the left ear. In cases of acute facial paralysis, the clinician must suspect herpes zoster oticus (Ramsay Hunt syndrome) and be vigilant for history or physical examination evidence of herpetic lesions of the ipsilateral pinna and/or ear canal (Figure 26-1). Sensorineural hearing loss is often seen in this disorder. Treatment of herpes zoster oticus is oral steroids and antiviral agents.

What do you do now?

Facial paralysis from acute otitis media (AOM)[2] carried an incidence of 0.5%–0.7% in the preantibiotic era; current incidence is 0.005%. It can affect all age groups, with a higher occurrence in younger children who develop AOM more frequently. The mechanism of facial paralysis is thought to be pressure and inflammation from the middle ear infection on the FN, which is not fully encased in a bony fallopian canal in the mastoid bone. The incidence of FN dehiscence in the temporal bone ranges from 20%–50%. Figure 26-2 demonstrates dehiscence and prolapse of the horizontal (middle ear) portion of the FN at the area of the oval window.

Facial paralysis from AOM is a surgical emergency and necessitates urgent release of the infectious pressure in the middle ear and, secondarily, on the FN in the fallopian canal. This is performed via a large myringotomy (incision in the tympanic membrane) with suction drainage of the middle ear fluid and placement of a large pressure-equalization tube to continue both drainage and subsequent aeration of the middle ear (Figure 26-3). When performed in a timely manner, complete resolution of the facial paralysis to a House-Brackmann grade 1 is to be expected in patients of all ages.[3]

TABLE 26-1 **House-Brackmann Facial Nerve Grading System**

Grade	Description
1	Normal function
2	Mild dysfunction, complete eye closure, normal symmetry at rest
3	Moderate dysfunction, complete eye closure, noticeable asymmetry at rest
4	Moderate-to-severe dysfunction, incomplete eye closure, obvious asymmetry
5	Severe dysfunction, incomplete eye closure, only twitch of gross motor movement
6	Total paralysis

Source: Nayak PK, Kumar RVS. Retromastoid-sub occipital: A novel approach to cerebello pontine angle in acoustic neuroma surgery-our experience in 21 cases. J Neurosci Rural Prac 2011;2:23–6.

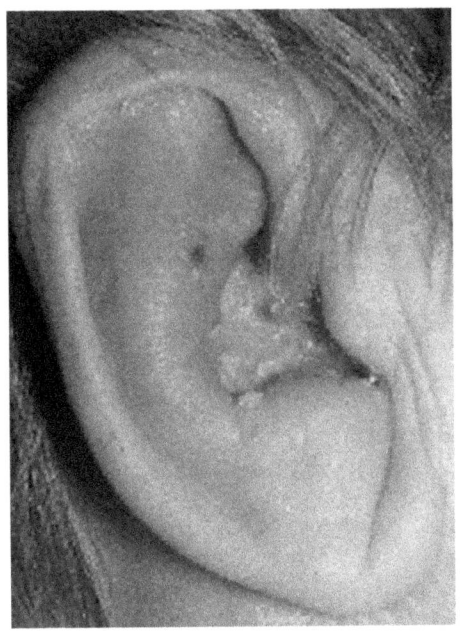

FIGURE 26-1 Herpes zoster oticus (Ramsay Hunt syndrome).

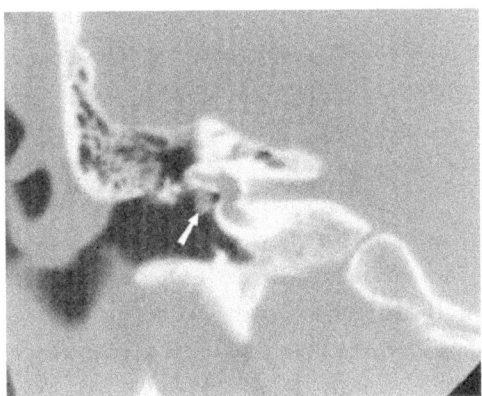

FIGURE 26-2 Facial nerve dehiscence in the horizontal fallopian canal. Source: Swartz JD, Harnsberger HR, Mukherji SK. The temporal bone. Radiol Clin North Am 1998;36:819–53.

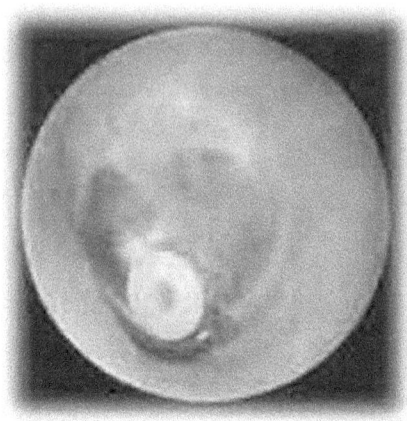

FIGURE 26-3 Myringotomy with pressure-equalization tube in place.

Chronic otitis media (COM) with or without presence of cholesteatoma can also cause facial paralysis. This often is seen in aggressive, untreated disease and requires mastoidectomy for removal of COM disease. Recovery of complete FN function in these cases is not as reliable.

FN paralysis that is identified immediately after ear surgery for otitis media is rare.[4] Deep injection of lidocaine into the anterior external auditory canal or near the mastoid tip can cause temporary weakness of the FN, which should resolve completely within 1–2 hours. Iatrogenic injury to the horizontal FN in an infected ear can occur in the presence of mucosal disease, including granulation tissue, in a patient with a bony dehiscence of the fallopian canal. The most common site of iatrogenic injury to the FN in ear surgery is inadvertent drilling into the second genu of the FN, between the horizontal and vertical segments. This is more common in badly diseased ears and sclerotic mastoids with poor pneumatization. The surgeon must be cognizant of the important landmarks to use to minimize risk to the FN. Use of intraoperative electrical monitoring may be helpful. Delayed FN paralysis after ear surgery is considered to be caused by local edema and may be accelerated by herpes simplex reactivation.

Acute facial paralysis from otitis media is an emergency.[5] Otolaryngologic evaluation and early, targeted intervention result in the best FN outcomes.

KEY POINTS TO REMEMBER

- FN weakness should be described using a commonly accepted scale, such as the six-point House-Brackmann grading scale, to allow for the most effective communication between health providers.
- Herpes zoster oticus (Ramsay Hunt syndrome) should be suspected in the patient with ear pain, vesicles on the pinna and/or ear canal, sensorineural hearing loss, and facial paralysis.
- FN paralysis in AOM is a surgical emergency and is treated with wide-field myringotomy, aspiration of middle ear fluid, and placement of a pressure-equalization tube, as well as other medical measures.
- Inadvertent administration of lidocaine near the FN may cause temporary, immediate FN paralysis, which resolves completely.
- The most common site for iatrogenic injury to the FN during COM surgery is drilling into the second surgical genu of the FN.
- Delayed FN paralysis after ear surgery is caused by local edema and may be accelerated by herpes simplex reactivation.

Further Reading

1. House JW, Brackmann DE. Facial nerve grading system. Otolaryngol Head Neck Surg 1985;93:146–7.
2. Gaio E, Marioni G, Tregnaghi A, Caltran S, Staffieri A. Facial nerve paralysis secondary to acute otitis media in infants and children. J Paediatr Child Health 2004;40:483–6.
3. Redaelli de Zinis LO, Gamba P, Balzanelli C. Acute otitis media and facial nerve paralysis in adults. Otol Neurotol 2003;24:113–7.
4. Wu W, Han D, Wang J, Yang W. [The observation of delayed facial paralysis after middle ear and mastoid surgery: 10 cases analysis.] Lin Chuang Er Bi Yan Hou Ke Za Zhi 2004;18:200–1.
5. Popovizer A, Raveh E, Bahar G, Oestreicher-Kedem Y, Feinmesser R, Nageris BI. Facial palsy associated with acute otitis media. Otolaryngol Head Neck Surg 2005;132:327–9.

27 Petrous Apicitis

A 23-year-old man presents with chronic drainage from his right ear and headache. He has double vision with right gaze. He has had no prior treatment. The drainage is described as thick and green. The headache is severe and is located behind his right eye. Past medical history is negative. Examination reveals a thin man with normal mental status. His left ear is normal; his right ear examination shows copious green drainage from a perforation in the tympanic membrane. He has erythema and edema in the right postauricular area. He has reactive right-sided cervical lymphadenopathy. Extraocular movement examination shows right lateral rectus palsy (Figure 27-1). Cranial nerve (CN) examination is also significant for right facial hypesthesia with reduced corneal reflex on the right. Facial nerve examination is normal. He has mixed hearing loss on the right.

What do you do now?

In the era of antibiotic treatment, petrous apicitis is a rare but life-threatening complication of otitis media. Classical findings include Gradenigo's triad of abducens palsy, retro-orbital pain, and suppurative otitis media. Ipsilateral trigeminal paresthesia is often seen. The pathophysiology is suppurative otitis media that affects the pneumatized space of the apex of the petrous pyramid. Adjacent to the inflamed apex are the abducens nerve (CN VI) in its canal (Dorello's canal), and the trigeminal nerve (CN V) ganglion. This is the cause of the diplopia, deep retro-orbital pain, and facial paresthesia.

Left untreated, petrous apicitis evolves into a more aggressive intracranial complication, including meningitis; cerebritis; intracranial abscess; spread to skull base with involvement of CN IX, X, XI (Vernet's syndrome); and spread to the prevertebral and parapharyngeal space and/or to the sympathetic plexus around the carotid artery.[1]

Diagnosis is confirmed by high-resolution computed tomography scan (Figure 27-2) of the temporal bone and magnetic resonance

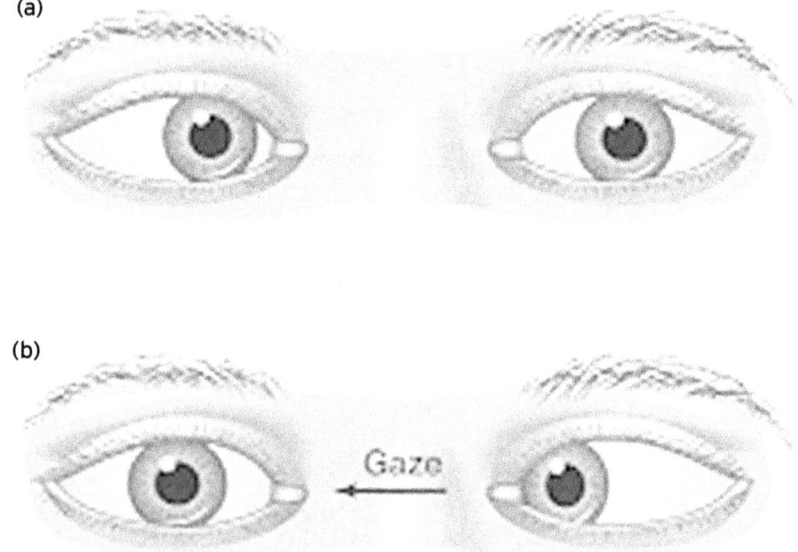

FIGURE 27-1 Right abducens nerve palsy. (a) Straight gaze. (b) Gaze to right. Note that right eye cannot move past midline to right, because of CN VI palsy.

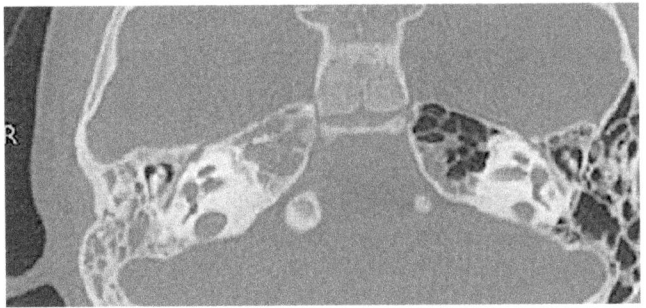

FIGURE 27-2 Axial temporal bone high-resolution computed tomography scan shows opacification of the pneumatized spaces of the right temporal bone, including mastoid air cells, middle ear cleft, and petrous apex. There is a small amount of air around only the epitympanic ossicles.[3]

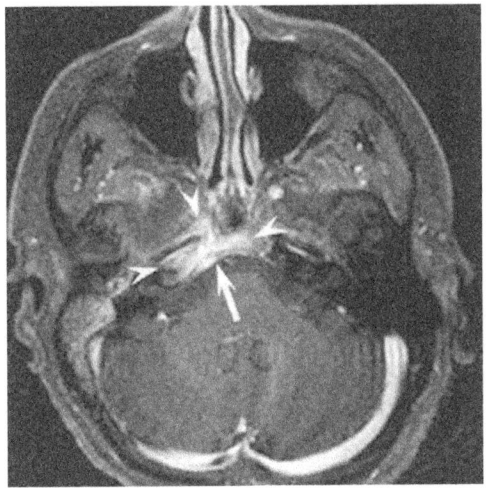

FIGURE 27-3 Axial contrast-enhanced T1-weighted magnetic resonance image shows abnormal enhancement throughout the right petrous apex (*arrowheads*), extending into the clivus and the region of Dorello's canal (*arrow*), and causing CN VI palsy.[4]

imaging (Figure 27-3), which are very useful in ruling out other intracranial extension or complication.

Treatment involves targeted intravenous antibiotics and surgical mastoidectomy with decompression and drainage of the petrous apex infection. There are cases where early identification led to the ability to treat this potential lethal problem with minimally invasive ventilation tube insertion.[2]

Early identification and treatment prior to development of significant intracranial and extracranial spread of infection carries the best prognosis.

> **KEY POINTS TO REMEMBER**
>
> - Gradenigo's triad in petrous apicitis is abducens (CN VI) palsy causing diplopia, retro-orbital pain, and suppurative otitis media, all occurring on the same side.
> - Ipsilateral facial paresthesia is often also seen, caused by CN V involvement.
> - Treatment includes intravenous antibiotics, mastoidectomy, and decompression and drainage of the petrous apex infection.
> - Left untreated, petrous apicitis evolves to include meningitis, cerebritis, intracranial abscess, and skull base spread with lower CN involvement, and may spread to the prevertebral or parapharyngeal spaces or the sympathetic plexus around the carotid artery.

Further Reading

1. Motamed M, Kalan A. Gradenigo's syndrome. Postgrad Med J 2000;76:559–60.
2. Kong SK, Lee IW, Goh EK, Park SE. Acute otitis media-induced petrous apicitis presenting as the Gradenigo syndrome: successfully treated by ventilation tube insertion. Am J Otolaryngol 2011;32:445–7.
3. Humayun H, Akhtar S, Ahmed, S. Gradenigo's syndrome–surgical management in a child. J Pakistan Med Assoc 2011;61(4):393–4.
4. Ahmad A, Branstetter BF. CT versus MR: still a tough decision. Otolaryngol Clin North Am 2008;41:1–22.

28 Meningitis and Brain Abscess

A 6-month-old baby girl is brought to the emergency room for lethargy and fever. She was in good health until the day prior, when she started to be "cranky" and have trouble drinking from the bottle. She now has a temperature of 102°F, has been vomiting, and is listless. Examination reveals acute otitis media (OM) in the left ear. She has nuchal rigidity and a positive Kernig's sign (pain with hip flexion to 90 degrees with knee extended) indicating at least meningism.[1]

What do you do now?

Fatigue, malaise, nuchal rigidity, and mental status changes are alarming findings in the pediatric or adult patient with OM. Meningitis is the most common intracranial complication of OM, and brain abscess is a particularly morbid complication, with a current mortality rate of 25%–41%. Incidence rates for meningitis and brain abscess secondary to OM vary widely, because the data[2] are based on small case reports and series, and often the distinction between acute and chronic OM is not made in the papers. Despite being in the era of antibiotic therapy, the rate of intracranial complications from OM is still approximately 8%, and is not limited to the developing world.[3,4] Published incidences of meningitis and cerebral abscess resulting from OM range from 6% to 44%.[5,6]

Workup involves laboratory analysis including complete blood count and erythrocyte sedimentation rate, often a lumbar puncture, and immediate head computed tomography scan and/or magnetic resonance imaging scan. The preformed pathways in the temporal bone between the aerated spaces and the subdural space remain open for at least 6 months after birth. These are conduits for direct intracranial extension. As such, the index of suspicion for an intracranial complication of acute OM in a small child should be very high. In older children and adults, otogenic brain abscesses are the result of venous thrombophlebitis rather than direct dural extension.

Immediate institution of broad-spectrum antibiotics and intravenous hydration is necessary.[7] Polymicrobial cultures with a high incidence of anaerobes are reported in cerebral abscesses from OM. Organisms include *Streptococcus, Staphylococcus, Escherichia coli, Proteus, Klebsiella*, and *Pseudomonas*, but, surprisingly, rarely *Haemophilus influenza*. Meningitis is managed with high-dose antibiotics, and possibly delayed myringotomy with tube insertion. Cerebral abscess often needs neurosurgical intervention for drainage. If the abscess is contiguous with the temporal bone, drainage may be accomplished by a temporal bone approach. This is of particular importance in brain abscesses from chronic OM.

Long-term sequelae of meningitis include permanent sensorineural hearing loss, from labyrinthitis that then develops into labyrinthitis ossificans. When sensorineural hearing loss is suspected, aggressive audiologic

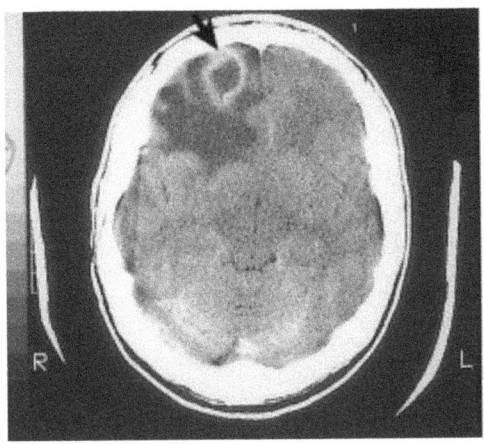

FIGURE 28-1 Single cerebral abscess (arrowhead) on computed tomography. Source: Spicer WJ. Clinical Microbiology and Infectious Diseases. Elsevier, Philadelphia, PA, 2008. pp. 102–3.

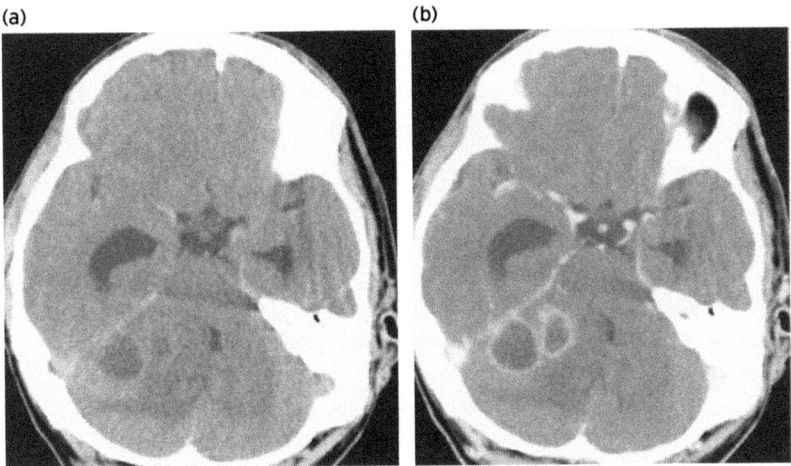

FIGURE 28-2 Cerebral abscesses in the posterior fossa after bacterial mastoiditis. (a) Noncontrast computed tomography shows a low-density lesion and perifocal edema in the right cerebellum, with compression of the fourth ventricle. (b) Contrast-enhanced computed tomography shows two ring-enhancing abscesses. Source: Thurnher MM. Meningitis and ventriculitis. In: Naidich TP, Castillo M, Cha S, Smirniotopoulos JG. Imaging of the Brain. Saunders, an imprint of Elsevier, Philadelphia, PA, 2013. pp. 865–76.

testing and early magnetic resonance imaging evaluation of the inner ear is necessary. Cochlear implantation hearing outcomes are significantly better in ears that are implanted before the ossification sets in, and this is a treatment priority (Figure 28-1 and Figure 28-2).[8]

Meningitis and otogenic brain abscesses are rare sequelae of acute and chronic OM. However, when present, the sequelae, including cranial nerve loss and death, can be devastating. Swift diagnosis and institution of effective treatment is critical.

> **KEY POINTS TO REMEMBER**
>
> - Meningitis is the most common intracranial complication of OM.
> - Brain abscess from OM carries a mortality rate of 25%–41%.
> - These complications from OM range in incidence from 6% to 44%, and are seen in both the developed and developing world.
> - Preformed pathways between the mastoid air cells and the subdural space remain open for 6 months after birth; infants with acute AOM should be considered at high risk for developing intracranial complication.
> - In addition to intravenous broad-spectrum antibiotics, otitic meningitis may be managed with myringotomy and tube insertion, and otogenic brain abscess needs drainage, preferably by a temporal bone approach.

Further Reading

1. [Guideline] Tunkel AR, Hartman BJ, Kaplan SL, Kaufman BA, Roos KL, Scheld WM, et al. Practice guidelines for the management of bacterial meningitis. Clin Infect Dis. Nov 1 2004;39(9):1267–84.
2. Geyik MF, Kokoglu OF, Hosoglu, Ayaz C. Acute bacterial meningitis as a complication of otitis media and related mortality factors. Yonsei Med J 2002:43:573–8.
3. Manzar N, Manzar B, Kumar R, Bari ME. The study of etiologic and demographic characteristics of intracranial brain abscess: a consecutive case series study from Pakistan. World Neurosurg 2011;76:195–200; discussion 79–83.
4. Gower D, McGuirt WF, Salem W. Intracranial complications of acute and chronic infections ear disease: a problem still with us. Laryngoscope 1983;93:1028–33.

5. Wanna GB, Dharamsi LM, Moss JR, Bennett ML, Thompson RC, Haynes DS. Contemporary management of intracranial complications of otitis media. Otol Neurotol 2009;31:111–7.
6. Penido NO, Borin A, Iha LCN, et al. Intracranial complications of otitis media: 15 years of experience in 33 patients. Otolaryngol Head Neck Surg 2005:132:37–42.
7. Mallur PS, Harirchian S, Lalwani AK. Preoperative and postoperative intracranial complications of acute mastoiditis. Ann Otol Rhinol Laryngol 2009;118:118–23.
8. Durisin M, Bartling S, Arnoldner C, et al. Cochlear osteoneogenesis after meningitis in cochlear implant patients: a retrospective analysis. Otol Neurotol 2010;31:1072–8.

29 Otitic Hydrocephalus

A five-year-old girl presented elsewhere with otorrhea through a pre-existing tympanostomy tube and partial ipsilateral facial palsy. Head computed tomography (CT) showed noncoalescent mastoiditis. Treatment with oral and topical antibiotics resulted in resolution of her facial palsy. Three weeks later, she presented to the emergency room with indolent headaches and vision changes. Examination revealed poor vision of 20/150 on the right and 20/80 on the left, bilateral sixth cranial nerve palsies, and severe optic nerve head swelling with associated hemorrhage. The original CT scan was reviewed and found to show sigmoid sinus thrombosis.[1]

What do you do now?

Given the extreme nature of the presentation, immediate lumbar puncture is indicated. When it demonstrates elevated cerebrospinal fluid (CSF) opening pressure, the diagnosis of otitic hydrocephalus is made. Treatment may include ventriculoperitoneal shunting, emergency mastoidectomy with removal of granulation tissue near the sigmoid sinus (but not necessarily removal of the thrombotic material), and intravenous antibiotics and anticoagulants. If the vision changes do not resolve promptly, optic nerve sheath fenestration may become necessary.

Otitic hydrocephalus, also referred to as pseudotumor cerebri, is an uncommon complication of otitis media. It is characterized by increased intracranial pressure without associated hydrocephalus. Patients present with headache, malaise, and vision changes. Papilledema and abducens palsy on ocular examination are common clinical findings. Four of 15 historical cases, and up to 25% of current cases, of pseudotumor cerebri reviewed had otitis media as their cause.[2,3]

The pathophysiology of otitic hydrocephalus remains controversial. Although some argue that involvement of the superior sagittal sinus by at least a mural thrombus is a necessary component of this

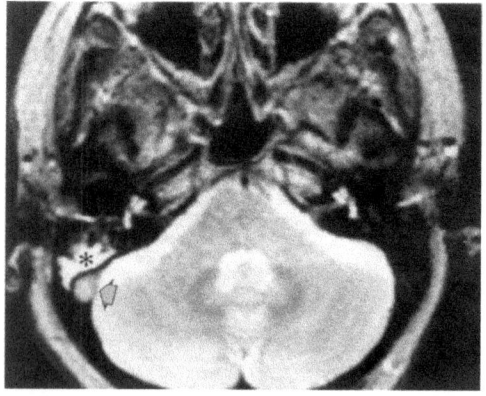

FIGURE 29-1 Axial postgadolinium T1-weighted magnetic resonance image. Hyperintense appearance in the left sigmoid sinus indicates thrombus (arrowhead). Asterisk shows a high signal area in the left temporal bone caused by chronic inflammatory process.[8]

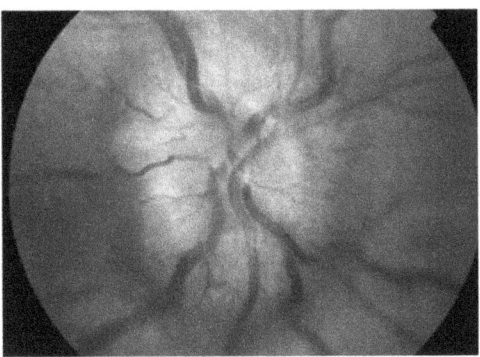

FIGURE 29-2 Papilledema in a 14 year old with hydrocephalus. Color photography shows a raised optic disc with blurred margins, filling of the cup, hyperemia, telangiectasia, vessel tortuosity and dilation, vessel obscuration by surrounding opaque retinal tissue, and disc and retinal hemorrhages. Disc telangiectasia is best seen in red-free images.

disease, there are case reports of otitic hydrocephalus without it.[4,5] The presence of thrombus in the lateral venous sinus alone may produce a rise in the cerebral venous pressure and a subsequent increase in CSF pressure.

Diagnosis is made, after a high index of suspicion, with imaging including CT of the head and magnetic resonance imaging scan (Figure 29-1). However, the definitive diagnosis is from elevated opening pressure with otherwise normal CSF examination on lumbar puncture. Ophthalmologic evaluation reveals papilledema (Figure 29-2).

Treatment options for this complication of otitis media are many. Medical treatment includes intravenous antibiotics and anticoagulants; diuretics, such as acetazolamide; and systemic steroids.[6] Surgical treatment includes mastoidectomy, decompression of thrombosed sinuses, and possibly optic sheath decompression and permanent ventriculoperitoneal shunting. In a review of 11 cases of pediatric otitic hydrocephalus, four were found to have post–otitis media occlusion of a lateral major sinus. Initial treatment with heparin followed by long-term acetylsalicylic acid led to complete recovery. Therefore, long-term anticoagulation, which is used in adults, is likely not necessary in children.[7]

KEY POINTS TO REMEMBER

- Otitic hydrocephalus is also called pseudotumor cerebri. A total of 25% of pseudotumor cerebri is caused by otitis media.
- It is characterized by increased intracranial pressure without hydrocephalus.
- Patients present with headache, malaise, and vision changes caused by papilledema and sixth cranial nerve (abducens nerve) palsy.
- Medical treatment includes intravenous antibiotics, anticoagulants, diuretics, and systemic corticosteroids.
- Surgical treatment includes mastoidectomy, decompression of thrombosed venous sinuses, possible optic sheath decompression, and permanent ventriculoperitoneal shunting.

Further Reading

1. Durairaj VD, Andrews B, Rao RR, Chan KH. Morbid complications of otitic hydrocephalus. Orbit 2008;27:51–4.
2. Bandyopadhyay S. Pseudotumor cerebri. Arch Neurol 2011;58:1699–701.
3. Davidoff LM. Pseudotumor cerebri: benign intracranial hypertension. Neurology 1956;6:605–15.
4. Tomkinson A, Mills RG, Cantrell PJ. The pathophysiology of otitic hydrocephalus. J Laryngol Otol 1997;111:757–9.
5. Kuczkowski J, Dubaniewicz-Wybieralska M, Przewozny T, Narozny W, Mikaszewski B. Otitic hydrocephalus associated with lateral sinus thrombosis and acute mastoiditis in children. Int J Pediatr Otol 2006;70:1817–23.
6. Isaacman DJ. Otitic hydrocephalus: an uncommon complication of a common condition. Ann Emerg Med 1989;18:684–7.
7. Reul J, Weber U, Kotlarek F, Isensee C, Thron A. [Cerebral vein and sinus thrombosis—an important cause of benign intracranial pressure increase in childhood.] Klin Paediatr 1997;209:116–20.
8. Sadhogi M, Dabirmoghaddam P. Otitic hydrocephalus: case report and literature review. Am J Otolaryngol 2007;28:187–90.

30 Lateral or Sigmoid Sinus Thrombosis

A 35-year-old woman presents with severe ear pain, intermittent fever, otorrhea, and headache for 5 days, worsening over time. She was treated for acute otitis media (AOM) starting 4 days prior by her primary care physician with oral antibiotics. She has a history of chronic ear disease for the past several months, and has had several courses of antibiotics as well as myringotomy and tube insertion. Examination reveals a septic-appearing woman with positive Griesinger sign[1] of tenderness and edema over the mastoid. She has no signs of papilledema.

What do you do now?

Lateral sinus and sigmoid sinus thrombosis are rare complications of otitis media (OM). Lateral sinus thrombosis (LST) accounts for 6% of all intracranial complications from OM in the era of antibiotic treatment. Prior to antibiotics, untreated OM with LST carried a 100% mortality rate. In the current era, LST is seen less commonly in children with acute OM and more often (although still rare) in adults with chronic OM and cholesteatoma.[2,3]

The classic finding in LST, which is from the preantibiotic era, is a "picket fence" fever curve. The variegations in fever are caused by periodic release of hemolytic streptococci from the septic sinus thrombus. When the sinus is completely occluded with thrombus, the blockage of cerebral venous outflow can go on to cause headache, papilledema, and increased intracranial pressure, as in otitic hydrocephalus.[4]

In the current era, the picket fence fever is rarely seen, and a high index of suspicion is necessary to make a timely diagnosis and institute proper intervention. The clinician should look for tenderness and edema over the mastoid, which are highly suggestive of LST and thrombosis of the mastoid emissary vein. If the thrombophlebitis extends into the jugular bulb and internal jugular vein, the patient may have neck pain with rotation or palpation. In severe cases of jugular bulb involvement, the patient may manifest Vernet's syndrome of paralysis of cranial nerves IX, X, and XI.[5]

In a retrospective review,[6] 100% of seven patients with LST secondary to OM presented with headache, otalgia, and AOM or otitis media with effusion (OME) on otoscopic examination. A total of 86% also had nausea and vomiting. Four patients had sixth cranial nerve palsy, whereas the following were present in three of the seven patients: dizziness, photophobia, anorexia, and fever within 24 hours. Two patients had blurry vision and papilledema.

In the current era, because chronic rather than acute OM is more likely the cause of LST, ear culture does not usually yield β-hemolytic streptococcus. Cultures usually show mixed flora. Blood cultures are generally negative, because the patient has commonly received antibiotics in the prodromal ear infection period.

Imaging studies include computed tomography (CT) scan with contrast that can show both the temporal bone pathology as well as a filling defect in the thrombosed sinus and a "delta sign" ring enhancement around the thrombosed area (Figure 30-1). Magnetic resonance imaging (MRI) is more sensitive than CT in detecting the thrombus (Figure 30-2). MRI and magnetic resonance venography can be used serially to examine clot progression and resolution (Figure 30-3).

Treatment of LST is with a combination of antibiotics and surgery. In selected early cases, intravenous antibiotics alone may be enough. In the past, anticoagulants were advocated to prevent extension of the thrombus distally; however, the infection is generally controllable with antibiotics and surgery, which accomplishes the same goal. Additionally, there is concern about risks of anticoagulants. The role of anticoagulants in the management of uncomplicated LST is still controversial.[7,8]

Surgical treatment is generally cortical mastoidectomy with removal of granulation tissue and/or cholesteatoma. The sigmoid sinus should be unroofed in this process. A needle is placed into the sinus. If free blood is aspirated, no further intervention is needed. If not, the sinus wall may be incised and the clot removed, but this step m Papilledema in a 14 year old with hydrocephalus. Color photography shows a raised optic disc with blurred margins, filling of the cup, hyperemia, telangiectasia, vessel tortuosity and dilation, vessel obscuration by surrounding opaque retinal tissue, and disc and retinal hemorrhages. Disc telangiectasia is best seen in red-free images. Papilledema in a 14 year old with hydrocephalus. Color photography shows a raised optic disc with blurred margins, filling of the cup, hyperemia, telangiectasia, vessel tortuosity and dilation, vessel obscuration by surrounding opaque retinal tissue, and disc and retinal hemorrhages. Disc telangiectasia is best seen in red-free images.

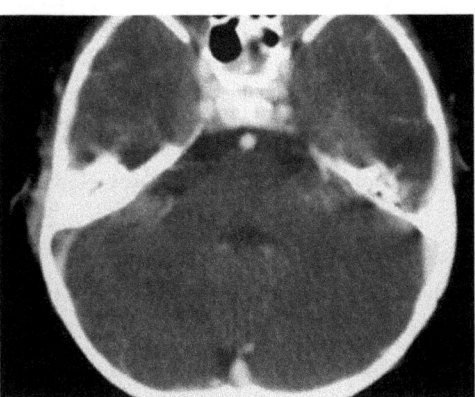

FIGURE 30-1 Posterior fossa CT venography on admission. A filling defect with high attenuation of the sinus walls (delta sign) is demonstrated in the right lateral sinus. On the left side is a normal-appearing sinus enhanced with contrast material.[10]

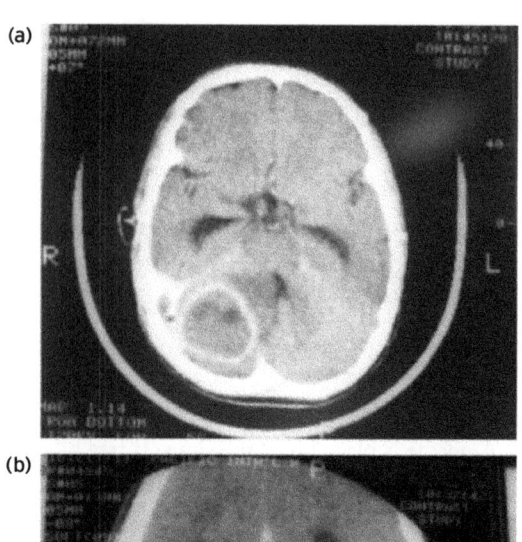

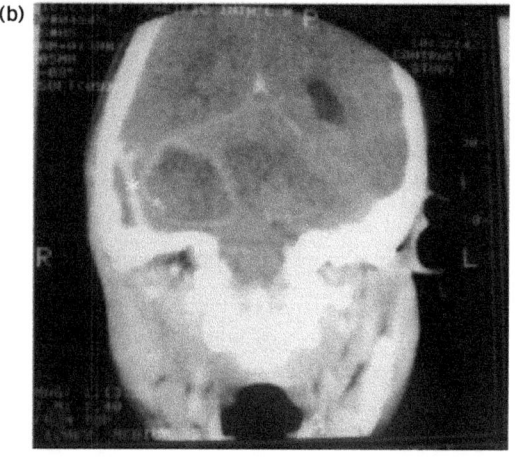

FIGURE 30-2 Photographs of the CT scans showing (a and b) cerebellar abscess of the right side with empty lateral sinus (delta sign) and the thickened dura and sinus wall (*) in between; tentorium is also visible in the coronal section (B).[11]

Papilledema in a 14 year old with hydrocephalus. Color photography shows a raised optic disc with blurred margins, filling of the cup, hyperemia, telangiectasia, vessel tortuosity and dilation, vessel obscuration by surrounding opaque retinal tissue, and disc and retinal hemorrhages. Disc telangiectasia is best seen in red-free images. ay also be unnecessary because there is evidence that the sinus recanalizes once the offending chronic OM is removed from the site. There is currently limited to no role for internal jugular vein ligation.

Postsurgically, the patient is maintained on intravenous antibiotics for 2–3 weeks, and serial MRI and magnetic resonance venography images

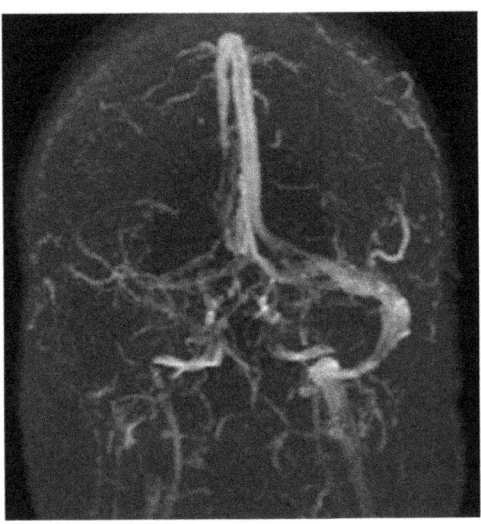

FIGURE 30-3 Magnetic resonance venography does not demonstrate any flow within the right transverse and sigmoid sinuses. Diagnosis: right transverse and sigmoid sinus thrombosis.[12]

should be performed to check for improvement as well as to rule out further intracranial complication.[9]

Without treatment, mortality is close to 100%. With treatment in the current era, it is less than 10%, and none in several series.

> **KEY POINTS TO REMEMBER**
>
> - "Picket fence" fever is rarely seen in the antibiotic era.
> - The patient may have headache, otalgia, AOM or OME, tenderness and edema over the mastoid bone, and neck pain with rotation or palpation. In severe cases, lower cranial nerve palsy may be present.
> - CT scan with intravenous contrast can show the pathognomic "delta sign" ring enhancement around the thrombosed lateral sinus. MRI may be more sensitive than CT in detecting the thrombus.
> - In early cases, intravenous antibiotics alone may be adequate treatment. The role of anticoagulants in uncomplicated LST is controversial. Surgery, when indicated, involves mastoidectomy, unroofing of the sigmoid sinus, and may or may not require thrombectomy.

Further Reading

1. Swartz J, Harsberger H, editors. Imaging of the Temporal Bone. 3rd edition. Thieme Publishers, New York, NY, 1998.
2. Bianchini C, Almoni C, Ceruti S, Grasso DL, Martini A. Lateral sinus thrombosis as a complication of acute mastoiditis. Acta Otorhinolaryngol Ital 2008;28:30–3.
3. Manolidis S, Kutz JW Jr. Diagnosis and management of lateral sinus thrombosis. Otol Neurotol 2005;26:1045–51.
4. Samuel J, Fernandes CM. Lateral sinus thrombosis: a review of 45 cases. J Laryngol Otol 1987;101:1227–9.
5. O'Connell JE. Lateral sinus thrombosis: a problem still with us. J Laryngol Otol 1990;104:949–51.
6. Christensen N, Wayman J, Spencer J. Lateral sinus thrombosis: a review of seven cases and proposal of a management algorithm. Int J Pediatr Otorhinolaryngol 2009;73:581–4.
7. Ropposch T, Nemetz U, Braun EM, Lackner A, Walch C. Low molecular weight heparin therapy in pediatric otogenic sigmoid sinus thrombosis: a safe treatment option? Int J Pediatr Otorhinolaryngol 2012;76:1023–6.
8. Bradley DT, Hashisaki GT, Mason JC. Otogenic sigmoid sinus thrombosis: what is the role of anticoagulation? Laryngoscope 2002;112:1726–9.
9. Ooi EH, Hilton M, Hunter G. Management of lateral sinus thrombosis: update and literature review. J Laryngol Otol 2003;117:932–9.
10. Tovi F, Hirsch M. Computed tomographic diagnosis of septic lateral sinus thrombosis. *The Annals of Otology, Rhinology & Laryngology* 1991;100(1):79–81.
11. Dubey SP. Intracranial spread of chronic middle ear suppuration. Am J Otolaryngol Head Neck Med Surg 31:73–7.
12. Fatterpekar GM. Teaching Files: Brain and Spine. Saunders, an imprint of Elsevier, Philadelphia, PA, 2012. pp. 172–3.

Index

Page numbers followed by *f* or *t* indicate figures or tables, respectively.

abducens nerve (CN VI), 208
abducens nerve (CN VI) lesions, 59*t*
abducens nerve (CN VI) palsy, 207, 208*f*, 210, 220
abscesses
 brain, 211–215
 cerebellar, 222–223, 223*f*
 cerebral, 212–214, 213*f*
Academy of Otolaryngology: guidelines for managing SSNHL, 15–17
acetylsalicylic acid, 30–31
acoustic neuroma, 40, 40*f*, 45–54, 48*f*, 51, 57
 growth rates, 46
 surgery for, 49
acoustic schwannoma, 53, 57
acute otitis media (AOM)
 complications of, 211, 212, 214, 221, 225
 facial paralysis from, 202, 204*f*, 205
acyclovir, 180
aging
 hearing loss associated with, 10
 progressive SNHL associated with, 3, 4, 4*f*
air-bone gap, 113, 114*f*, 117
Albers-Schönberg disease, 172*t*, 173
Alport syndrome, 36*t*
American Academy of Otolaryngology-Head and Neck Surgery Foundation: diagnostic criteria for Ménière's disease, 67, 68*t*
aminoglycosides, 28, 29–30, 29*t*
antibiotics
 aminoglycoside, 28, 29–30, 29*t*
 macrolide, 31
 ototoxicity, 31

antineoplastics, 31
antiviral agents, 180
Antoni A, 46
Antoni B, 46
AOM. *See* acute otitis media
arachnoid cysts, 58
arteriovenous fistulas (AVFs), 154–155, 154*f*, 157
arteriovenous malformations (AVMs), 152, 153*f*
 key points to remember, 157
 temporal lobe, 152, 153*f*, 157
audiometric evaluation, normal, 75, 76*f*
autoimmune labyrinthitis, 84
autoimmune lesions, 58, 59*t*
AVFs. *See* arteriovenous fistulas
AVMs. *See* arteriovenous malformations
axonotmesis, 170, 170*t*

bacterial labyrinthitis, 84, 85*t*
bacterial mastoiditis, 212–214, 213*f*
behavioral treatment, 139
Bell's palsy, 175–182
 House-Brackmann grading scale for, 177, 178*t*, 201, 202*t*
 recurrent, 193, 194*f*, 195*f*, 196, 197*f*
benign intracranial hypertension (BIH), 159–162, 160*f*
benign paroxysmal positional vertigo (BPPV), 91–96
BIH. *See* benign intracranial hypertension
bilateral sudden hearing loss, 14–15
blunt temporal bone trauma, 185–190
boat-like vertigo, 102
bone-anchored hearing aids, 7, 8*f*
bone conduction devices, 7, 8*f*
bony fallopian canal: facial nerve dehiscence in, 202, 203*f*

BPPV. *See* benign paroxysmal positional vertigo
brain abscesses, 211–215
brain neoplasms, 58
brainstem lesions, 59*t*
branchio-oto-renal syndrome, 37*t*
buccal nerve, 171*t*

carotid-cavernous fistula (CCF), 155, 157
cerebellar abscesses, 222–223, 223*f*
cerebellar lesions, 59*t*
cerebellopontine angle tumors, 40, 40*f*, 45–54
　key points to remember, 53, 60
　rare tumors, 55–61, 56*f*, 57*f*, 59*t*
cerebral abscesses, 212–214, 213*f*
cervical nerve, 171*t*
CHARGE syndrome, 172*t*, 173
chemotherapy, 28, 29*t*, 31
chorda tympani, 171*t*
chromosome 22q11.2 deletion syndrome, 172*t*, 173
chronic otitis media (COM), 204, 205, 212
cinchonism, 31
clonazepam, 139
cochlear implants, 7–10, 9*f*
cochlin-tomoprotein testing, 109
cognitive behavioral treatment, 139
computed tomography (CT), high-resolution, 208–209, 209*f*
concussion, labyrinthine, 123–129
conductive hearing loss, 117
conductive hyperacusis, 117
congenital facial palsy, 169–174
　classification of, 170, 170*t*
　familial, 172*t*, 173
　nontraumatic etiology of, 172*t*, 173
congenital hearing loss, 33–38
congenital rest-associated lesions, 59*t*
congenital rests, intracranial, 59*t*
congenital unilateral lower lip palsy, 172*t*, 173

corticosteroids, 180
cranial nerve VI (abducens nerve), 208
cranial nerve VI (abducens nerve) lesions, 59*t*
cranial nerve VI (abducens nerve) palsy, 207, 208*f*, 210, 220
CT. *See* computed tomography
Cyber Knife, 48
cysts, arachnoid, 58

Dandy diagnostic criteria, 160–161
dehiscence
　facial nerve, 202, 203*f*
　superior semicircular canal, 113–121, 164, 165, 165*f*
　tegmen, 163–166, 164*f*, 165*f*
delayed facial nerve palsy, 189
delayed facial nerve paralysis, 205
delta sign, 221, 222*f*, 223*f*, 225
dexamethasone, 16
DFNA, 34
DFNB, 34
diet, 138
disc telangiectasia, 223, 224
diuretics
　loop, 28, 29*t*, 30
　ototoxicity, 28, 29*t*, 30
Dix-Hallpike maneuver, 93, 93*f*
Dorello's canal, 208
drugs, ototoxic, 28, 29*t*, 31, 32
dysequilibrium, 65–129
dysgeusia, 176

ear trauma, penetrating, 105, 106*f*
effusions: otitis media with, 221
electrocochleography, 70
electromyography, voluntary, 190
electroneuronography (ENOG), 189
electrophysiologic studies, 189–190
empty sella, 160*f*, 161
endolymphatic hydrops, idiopathic, 66
ENOG. *See* electroneuronography
epidermoids, 56–57, 56*f*, 57*f*

epiphora, 176
Epley maneuver, 93, 94f
erythromycin, 28, 29t, 31

facial nerve (FN) branches, 171t
facial nerve (FN) dehiscence, 202, 203f
facial nerve (FN) injury, 170, 170t, 184
facial nerve (FN) palsy
  congenital, 169–174
  delayed, 189
  traumatic, 183–192
facial nerve (FN) schwannomas, 60, 194
  diagnostic evaluation of, 196
  differential diagnosis of, 195–196
  symptoms of, 195
  treatment of, 197, 198
facial nerve (FN) weakness: House-Brackmann grading scale for, 177, 178t, 201, 202t
facial neuroma, 193–198, 197f
facial neuropathy, 169–198
facial paralysis
  delayed, 205
  from otitis media, 201–205, 202, 204f
  recurrent, 193, 194f, 195f, 196, 197f
  unilateral, 177, 179t
facial paresis, idiopathic, 176
facioscapulohumeral muscular dystrophy, 172t, 173
fallopian canal: facial nerve dehiscence in, 202, 203f
famciclovir, 180
familial congenital facial palsy, 172t, 173
fever, "picket fence," 221, 225
Fisch Classification System, 147
fistulas
  arteriovenous, 154–155, 154f, 157
  carotid-cavernous, 155, 157
  perilymphatic, 105–111
FN. *See* facial nerve

fractures, temporal bone, 185–186, 186–188, 186f, 187f, 188f
furosemide testing, 69–70

Gamma Knife radiation, 48–49
GJ tumors. *See* glomus jugulare tumors
Glasscock-Jackson classification
  for GJ tumors, 147
  for GT tumors, 145–147
glomus jugulare (GJ) tumors, 144–145, 146f, 147, 147f, 148
  case history, 148–149
  key points to remember, 149
glomus tumors, 144, 147
glomus tympanicum (GT) tumors, 144, 145–147, 145f, 149
glycerol testing, 69–70
Goldenhar syndrome, 172t, 173
Gradenigo's triad, 208, 210
greater superficial petrosal nerve, 171t
GT tumors. *See* glomus tympanicum tumors

head trauma, 128
hearing aids, 139–140
hearing conservation, 23–24, 24–25
hearing loss (HL), 1–61
  associated with aging, 10
  asymmetric, 27, 28f
  conductive, 117
  congenital, 33–38
  hereditary, 34–35, 34t, 36t–37t
  key points to remember, 10
  noise-induced, 21–26, 22f, 23f, 134, 136, 137f
  progressive, 15
  sensorineural, 3, 4, 4f, 13–19
  sudden, 14
hemifacial microsomia, 172t, 173
Hennebert's sign, 116, 126
hereditary hearing loss (HHL), 34–35
  inheritance patterns, 34, 34t
  syndromic, 35, 36t–37t
herpes zoster oticus, 201, 203f, 205

HHL. *See* hereditary hearing loss
HL. *See* hearing loss
House-Brackmann grading scale, 177, 178*t*, 201, 202*t*
hydrocephalus, otitic, 217–220, 218*f*, 219*f*
hyperacusis, 117, 176
hypertension, intracranial
  benign, 159–162, 160*f*
  idiopathic, 160

idiopathic facial paresis, 176
idiopathic intracranial hypertension, 160
implantable hearing processors, 7, 8*f*
inflammatory lesions, 58, 59*t*
injury
  facial nerve, 170, 170*t*, 184
  temporal bone, 183, 184*f*
internal carotid artery, aberrant, 156*f*, 157
intracranial congenital rests, 59*t*
intracranial hypertension
  benign, 159–162, 160*f*
  idiopathic, 160
intracranial lipomas, 58, 59*t*
intrauterine misoprostol exposure, 172*t*, 173
intrauterine thalidomide exposure, 172*t*, 173

Jacobson nerve, 145*f*
JBAs. *See* jugular bulb anomalies
Jervell and Lange-Nielsen syndrome, 37*t*
jugular bulb anomalies (JBAs), 155, 156*f*, 157
jugulotympanic paragangliomas, 144

Kernig's sign, 211

labyrinthine concussion, 123–129
labyrinthitis, 83–89
  bacterial, 84, 85*t*
  pathogens that cause, 84–85, 85*t*
  viral, 84, 85*t*

lateral sinus thrombosis (LST), 221–226, 222*f*
Lempert supine roll maneuver, 93
Lermoyez attacks, 67–68
lipoma, intracranial, 58
loop diuretics, 28, 29*t*, 30
lower lip palsy, congenital unilateral, 172*t*, 173

macrolides, 31
magnetic resonance imaging, 208–209, 209*f*
  gadolinium-enhanced, 136
marginal mandibular nerve, 171*t*
masking devices, ear-level, 139–140
medical treatment, 139
Ménière's disease, 65–74, 66*f*
  diagnostic criteria for, 67, 68*t*
  differential diagnosis of, 70, 71*t*
Meniette device, 71–72
meningioma, 51–52, 52*t*, 53*f*, 57
meningitis, 211–215
meningoencephalocele, 164, 164*f*, 165*f*
metastatic lesions, 59*t*
microsomia, hemifacial, 172*t*, 173
middle fossa approach repair, 118–119
migraine, vestibular, 98
migraine-associated vertigo, 102
migrainous vertigo, 97–104, 100*t*
misoprostol exposure, intrauterine, 172*t*, 173
Möbius syndrome, 172*t*, 173
muscular dystrophy, facioscapulohumeral, 172*t*, 173
myringotomy, 202, 204*f*

nerve damage, 21, 33
nerve excitability testing, 190
nervus intermedius (Wrisberg nerve), 171*t*
neurofibromatosis (NF), 39–43, 40*f*
neurofibromatosis 1 (NF1), 41, 43
neurofibromatosis 2 (NF2), 37*t*, 41, 42, 43, 46

neuroma
  acoustic, 40, 40f, 45–54, 48f, 51, 57
  facial, 193–198, 197f
Neuromonics™ tinnitus treatment device, 139–140
neuropraxia, 170, 170t
neurotmesis, 170, 170t
NIHL. *See* noise-induced hearing loss
noise exposure
  permissible, 23, 24t
  in workplace, 23, 24t
noise-induced hearing loss (NIHL), 21–26, 22f, 23f, 136
  asymmetric, 134, 137f
  key points to remember, 26
noisy work environments, 23–24

Occupational Safety and Health Administration (OSHA)
  requirements for hearing conservation, 24–25
  requirements for hearing conservation in noisy work environments, 23–24
ophthalmalgia, 176
optic nerve abnormalities, 160f, 161
otalgia, 176
otic capsule, 186–187, 187f
otic capsule–violating temporal bone fractures, 186–188, 188f
otitic hydrocephalus, 217–220, 218f, 219f
otitis media (OM)
  acute, 202, 204f, 205, 211, 212, 214, 221, 225
  chronic, 204, 205, 212
  complications of, 201–226
  facial paralysis from, 201–205
otitis media with effusion (OME), 221
ototoxic drugs, 28, 29t, 31, 32
ototoxicity, 28, 32
ototoxins, 27–32, 139

palsy
  abducens nerve (CN VI), 207, 208f, 210, 220
  Bell's palsy, 175–182
  facial, 169–174, 183–192
papilledema, 219, 219f, 223, 224
paragangliomas, 143–150
paralysis, facial, 201–205
  from acute otitis media, 202, 204f
  from chronic otitis media, 204
  delayed, 205
  recurrent, 193, 194f, 195f, 196, 197f
  unilateral, 177, 179t
paresis, facial, 176
Pendred syndrome, 36t
penetrating ear trauma, 105, 106f
penetrating temporal bone trauma, 184–185
perilymphatic fistula, 105–111
peripheral neurofibromatosis, 41
peripheral vertigo, 79, 79f
petrous apicitis, 207–210, 209f
"picket fence" fever, 221, 225
pneumolabyrinth, 108–109, 108f
polyarteritis nodosa, 84
posterior fossa: cerebral abscesses after bacterial mastoiditis in, 212–214, 213f
prednisone
  for Bell's palsy, 180
  for idiopathic SSNHL, 16
presbycusis, 3–11, 4f
  characteristics of hearing loss in, 5–6, 5t
  types of, 5–6, 5t
pressure-induced vertigo, 113, 114f
pseudotumor cerebri, 160f, 161, 218, 220
pulsatile tinnitus, 151, 157
  right-sided, 163
  treatment of, 161

quality of life, 134
quinine, 28, 29t, 31, 138

radiation therapy, 48–49
Ramsay Hunt syndrome, 177, 201, 203f, 205
rare tumors, 55–61, 56f, 57f, 59t
Recklinghausen disease, 41
round window occlusion, 119

salicylates, 28, 29t
schwannomas
  acoustic, 53, 57
  facial, 60, 194, 195–196, 197, 198
  vestibular, 41, 42f, 45–51, 48f, 53, 57
sella, empty, 160f, 161
sensorineural hearing loss (SNHL)
  asymmetric, 83, 84f, 193, 194f
  mild-to-moderate, 105, 106f
  profound, 39, 40f
  progressive, 3, 4, 4f
  sudden, 13–19, 14f
serous labyrinthitis, 84–85
SHL. *See* sudden hearing loss
sigmoid sinus thrombosis, 217, 218f, 221–226, 224f
skull-based neoplasms, 59t, 60
SNHL. *See* sensorineural hearing loss
Sophono system, 7, 9f
SoundBite devices, 7, 8f
sound-induced vertigo, 113, 114f
Spetzler-Marlin grading, 152
SSCD. *See* superior semicircular canal dehiscence
SSNHL. *See* sudden sensorineural hearing loss
stereotactic irradiation (SI), 48–49
Stickler syndrome, 37t
sudden hearing loss (SHL)
  bilateral, 14–15
  definition of, 14
sudden sensorineural hearing loss (SSNHL), 13–19, 14f
superior semicircular canal dehiscence (SSCD), 113–121, 115f, 164, 165f

  clinical presentation of, 116
  diagnostic evaluation of, 116–118
  hallmark symptoms, 120
  key points to remember, 120, 165
  treatment of, 118–119
superior semicircular canal resurfacing or plugging, 118–119
suppurative labyrinthitis, 84
surgery
  for superior semicircular canal dehiscence, 118–119
  for vestibular schwannoma, 49, 50
swaying, 102

tegmen dehiscence (TD), 163–166, 164f, 165f
temporal bone, 208–209, 209f
temporal bone fractures
  longitudinal, 185–186, 186f
  oblique, 186, 187f
  otic capsule–sparing, 186–188, 188f
  otic capsule–violating, 186–188, 188f
  transverse, 185–186, 186f
temporal bone trauma
  blunt, 185–190
  penetrating, 183, 184–185, 184f
temporal lobe arteriovenous malformations, 152, 153f, 157
thalidomide exposure, intrauterine, 172t, 173
thrombosis
  lateral or sigmoid sinus, 221–226, 222f
  sigmoid sinus, 217, 218f, 224f
tinnitus, 23–24, 65, 66f, 133–166
  causes of, 134
  key points to remember, 140
  pulsatile, 151, 157, 161, 163
  subjective, 133–142
  treatment considerations, 138–140
Tinnitus Handicap Inventory, 134, 135t–136t
tinnitus therapy, 25

toxins, 27–32
transcanal approach, 119
transmastoid approach, 119
transverse sinus stenosis, 160f, 161
trauma
    blunt temporal bone, 185–190
    head, 128
    penetrating ear, 105, 106f
    penetrating temporal bone, 183, 184–185, 184f
    vertigo after, 105, 106f, 128
traumatic facial palsy, 183–192
Treacher Collins syndrome, 37t
Tullio phenomenon, 116, 126
tumors
    cerebellopontine angle, 40, 40f, 45–54, 55–61
    glomus, 144, 147
    glomus jugulare (GJ), 144–145, 146f, 147, 147f, 148–149
    glomus tympanicum (GT), 144, 145–147, 145f, 149

unilateral facial paralysis, 177, 179t
unilateral lower lip palsy, congenital, 172t, 173
Usher syndrome, 36t

valacyclovir, 180
Valsalva maneuver, 116–117
vancomycin, 28, 29t
vascular lesions, 59t, 60
vasculature, aberrant, 155–157
Vernet's syndrome, 208
vertigo, 65–129
    benign paroxysmal positional, 91–96
    boat-like, 102
    continuous, 75, 76f
    episodic, 65, 66f, 69

    after head trauma, 128
    migraine-associated, 102
    migrainous, 97–104
    after penetrating ear trauma, 105, 106f
    peripheral, 79, 79f
    sound-induced, 113, 114f
    unremitting, 83, 84f
vestibular Ménière's disease, 67
vestibular migraine, 98
vestibular neuronitis, 76
    clinical presentation of, 77
    diagnosis of, 77
    diagnostic evaluation of, 77–79
    differential diagnosis of, 78–79
    natural history of, 79–80
    symptoms of, 77
    treatment of, 80
vestibular neuropathy, 75–82
vestibular schwannoma (VS), 45–51, 48f, 57
    bilateral, 41, 42f
    key points to remember, 53
vestibular therapy, 80, 94
Vibrant floating mass transducers, 7, 8f
viral labyrinthitis, 84, 85t
VS. *See* vestibular schwannoma

Waardenburg syndrome, 36t
Wegener's granulomatosis, 84
workplace
    permissible noise exposure in, 23, 24t
    requirements for hearing conservation in, 23–24, 24–25
Wrisberg nerve (nervus intermedius), 171t

xerophthalmia, 176
xerostomia, 176

zygomatic nerve, 171t

www.ingramcontent.com/pod-product-compliance
Ingram Content Group UK Ltd.
Pitfield, Milton Keynes, MK11 3LW, UK
UKHW021302180426
11947UKWH00015B/970